PRAISE FOR

The New
McDOUGALL
COOKBOOK

"John and Mary McDougall are reaching millions of people with information that can be life-saving. This book shows how food can be both delicious *and* nutritious."

> —Dean Ornish, M.D., president and director,
> Preventative Medicine Research Institute;
> author of *Dr. Dean Ornish's Program for
> Reversing Heart Disease*

"Scientific understanding of good nutrition is but one step; putting it into practice is quite another. John and Mary McDougall have done both."

> —T. Colin Campbell, professor and director,
> China-Oxford-Cornell Diet, Lifestyle, and
> Nutrition Project, Cornell University;
> and Karen Campbell

JOHN AND MARY MCDOUGALL live in Santa Rosa, California, where John runs a nationally renowned in-patient program at St. Helena Hospital and Mary teaches health-promoting cooking. In addition to their books, they have recently launched McDougall's Right Foods™, featuring prepackaged healthy instant meals.

The New
McDOUGALL
COOKBOOK

John McDougall, M.D., and Mary McDougall

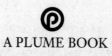

A PLUME BOOK

PUBLISHER'S NOTE
The ideas, procedures, and suggestions contained in this book
are not intended as a substitute for consulting with your physician.
All matters regarding your health require medical supervision.

PLUME
Published by the Penguin Group
Penguin Books USA Inc., 375 Hudson Street, New York, New York 10014, U.S.A.
Penguin Books Ltd, 27 Wrights Lane, London W8 5TZ, England
Penguin Books Australia Ltd, Ringwood, Victoria, Australia
Penguin Books Canada Ltd, 10 Alcorn Avenue, Toronto, Ontario, Canada M4V 3B2
Penguin Books (N.Z.) Ltd, 182–190 Wairau Road, Auckland 10, New Zealand

Penguin Books Ltd, Registered Offices: Harmondsworth, Middlesex, England

Published by Plume, an imprint of Dutton Signet,
a division of Penguin Books USA Inc.
Previously published in a Dutton edition.

First Plume Printing, January, 1997
10 9 8 7 6 5 4 3 2 1

 REGISTERED TRADEMARK—MARCA REGISTRADA

The Library of Congress has catalogued the Dutton edition as follows:

McDougall, John A.
    The new McDougall cookbook / John McDougall and Mary McDougall
        p.   cm.
    Includes index.
    ISBN 0-525-93610-6 (hc.)
    ISBN 0-452-27465-6 (pbk.)
    1. Low-fat diet—Recipes.   2. Vegetarian cookery.   I. McDougall,
Mary A. (Mary Ann)   II. Title.
RM237.7.M42   1993
641.5'638—dc20   92–41041
                                                          CIP

Printed in the United States of America
Original hardcover design by Eve L. Kirch

CONTENTS

The New
McDOUGALL
COOKBOOK

INTRODUCTION: THE McDOUGALL QUICK START PROGRAM

Many of you don't have the time to read through a 350-page book on diet and health before you change your way of eating. The first two chapters offer the essence of the McDougall Program diet, presented more concisely than ever before. Close to 350 of Mary McDougall's recipes and contributions of faithful followers of the McDougall Program follow this short introduction. These creations mark a tremendous jump forward in creativity and tastiness. Also included is an updated "Canned and Packaged Products List." You and your family will be introduced to some of the best-tasting food you've ever enjoyed, and the changes you will see in your health and appearance will very much reward the efforts you will make to alter your eating habits.

Medical Care

Many people turn to the McDougall Program for medical reasons, and, of course, one of the goals of the program is to get peo-

1

ple off medication. One of the comforts gained by the patients who attend my program at St. Helena Hospital and Health Center is medical supervision. Within the first few days most have stopped taking all pills for controlling diabetes and high blood pressure; some have stopped taking all insulin and heart medications. All of this is done under the guidance of a physician familiar with the effects of diet and exercise on health and medication needs.

If you are actually sick or taking medication, I strongly urge you to find such a doctor to help you make important medical decisions. Changes in diet and lifestyle can be very powerful. And unless medication dosages are reduced properly over a period of time, you could experience adverse effects. Furthermore, any disease requires correct diagnosis, and many people need more help than a healthful diet and lifestyle alone can provide. So make the effort to achieve a doctor-patient relationship that is productive and pleasant.

Times are changing, happily, and nowadays many more doctors are realizing the importance of good nutrition for health and healing. Your improvement may be just the kind of instruction your doctor needs to stimulate further interest in the subject and to treat patients with similar problems.

Nutritional Adequacy

A starch-based diet with the addition of fruits and vegetables as recommended in the McDougall Program is ideal nutrition for adults and children over the age of two years. All of your needs for protein, essential amino acids, essential fats, carbohydrates, minerals, and vitamins are supplied in optimal amounts for growth and maintenance. Requirements for vitamin B_{12} may be the only exception. Very rare cases of B_{12} deficiency have been found in strict vegetarians. To guard against this risk, you should take 5 mcg (micrograms) of B_{12} per day if you are pregnant or nursing, or have been on the Program without other reliable sources of B_{12} for more than three years.

Human breast milk exclusively is the ideal nutrition for the first six months of life. Infant formulas are a poor substitute. Starches and fruits (and some vegetables) are added at about six months, but breast milk (or a substitute) is continued until at least two years. Most children tolerate high-fat plant foods, such as nuts (e.g., in the form of peanut butter), seeds, olives, avocados, and soybeans (e.g., in the form of tofu), well, and many can use the extra fat and calories.

Program Modifications

Variations in the Program are occasionally made for individuals. Common diet modifications include the following:

- For faster weight loss, all flour products (breads, bagels, pastas, etc.) are eliminated, and green and yellow vegetable intake is increased.
- For weight gain, flour products are emphasized, dried fruits are added, and high-fat plant foods sometimes make up a larger than usual part of the diet.
- Indigestion (gastritis) sometimes requires the elimination of raw vegetables (especially onions, green peppers, cucumbers, and radishes), fruit juices, and hot sauces.
- In general, legumes (beans, peas, and lentils) should be limited to 1 cooked cup per day because of their high protein content.
- Protein from beans, peas, and lentils is severely restricted in patients with kidney and liver failure, kidney stones, gout, and osteoporosis.
- In general, fruits should be limited to three servings per day because of the simple sugars.
- All simple sugars (especially those from fruit and fruit juice) are restricted for those with elevated blood triglycerides.
- Foods causing adverse reactions, such as allergies, to individuals are removed from the diet. For details on nutrition and medical issues, refer to previous McDougall books, like *The McDougall Plan* (New Win Publishing Inc.), *McDougall's Medicine* (New Win Publishing Inc.), and *The McDougall Program* (Plume Books).

CHAPTER 1

McDOUGALLING

The McDougall Philosophy

People all over the Western world are talking about lowering their fat, cholesterol, and salt intake by eating less meat, dairy products, eggs, and processed foods, and by increasing their consumption of complex carbohydrates and fiber by eating more whole grains, fresh fruits, and vegetables. Even with the best of intentions, though, many of these people will fall short of the ideal of healthful eating unless they follow the principles of the McDougall Program.

During my two decades of medical practice, I have heard many people complain about the diet books they have read, the cooking classes and health resorts they have attended, and the "healthy heart" studies in which they have participated. Each endeavor ended in common disappointments: improvements in health and appearance were minimal and temporary. Most demanded a super-human willpower to endure hunger all day, every day, and some prescribed medications.

Your expectations for an effective, safe, and easy health program will be fulfilled only when you accept the need for a starch-based meal plan and daily exercise. Ours is a practical program that works, because there are no restrictions on the *amount* of recommended foods you can eat. In a short time you will love the tastes of healthful foods and the good feelings that are generated by exercise. Most people who really learn the principles of the McDougall Program easily remain faithful to it.

You don't have to be a medical genius to realize that limiting your intake of rich foods will prevent poor health. The most powerful medicine in the Western world is the knowledge that removing these burdensome foods from a sick person's diet will help him or her to recover. Daniel described in the Bible 2,500 years ago the poor health of his men living in the king's palace. When they switched from eating the "royal food" to vegetables and water, their health improved within ten days.

> Daniel then said to the guard whom the chief official had appointed over Daniel, Mishael, and Azariah, "Please test your servants for ten days: Give us nothing but vegetables to eat and water to drink. Then compare our appearance with that of the young men who eat the royal food, and treat your servants in accordance with what you see." So he agreed to this and tested them for ten days.
>
> At the end of the ten days they looked healthier and better nourished than any of the young men who ate the royal food. (Dan. 1:11–15; Holy Bible, New International Version.)

The natural-hygiene movement in the United States of the early nineteenth century identified the importances of a vegetarian diet and a wholesome lifestyle for health and healing. Today, people following the teachings of Walter Kempner, M.D., Michio Kushi (macrobiotics), Dean Ornish, M.D., and Nathan Pritikin, to name only a few of the more recent proponents, realize the miraculous healing power of proper diet and lifestyle. All of these approaches share a starch-based diet, moderate exercise, and good health habits as their basis for treatment.

Many programs advocate a low-fat, low-cholesterol, high-carbohydrate, high-fiber diet and adequate exercise as the path to good health and lifelong weight loss. I would not object to your following any of them. The differences between the various programs that use this general approach to health and healing are minimal. These details are more important in the effects they have on your acceptance and continued adherence to the program than on the actual improvements in health and appearance they can achieve. Of all these approaches, the McDougall Program presents the easiest and most effective one for several important reasons.

The All-American Way

Recipes in some other low-fat cookbooks are difficult to accept because they call for ingredients unfamiliar to most Americans. Some writers recommend raw ingredients and cumbersome rules for serving them in combinations. Even more foreign are the macrobiotic teachings, which rely on Oriental ingredients that are common to Japanese people but are not generally found in American supermarkets.

The McDougall Program is based on *familiar* ingredients and on simple and consistent methods of preparation. When you understand these basic principles, you can try different ways of balancing and/or combining foods. These methods, while they may sometimes be inconvenient, are not harmful.

A Moderate Approach

If you are familiar with the McDougall Program, you probably haven't thought of it as being moderate. If you consider our system stringent, however, you need only look into the Kempner Diet used at Duke University Medical School to get another perspective. Walter Kempner, M.D., begins by feeding his patients limited amounts of white rice and fruit. That's all. Later on, as their health improves, they are given some vegetables, and, if recovery goes well, they will eventually be allowed small amounts of lean meat. Now that's a spartan regimen!

In the other direction, the Pritikin Program is more lenient than ours. Nathan Pritikin allowed small amounts of lean beef, chicken, and fish, and low-fat dairy products in his program. He told me that these animal foods were included because he believed they would make the meal plan more acceptable to people, although he understood from scientific research that they were not essential for good nutrition. The McDougall Program takes a middle course.

The McDougall Program is based on common starches, such as oatmeal, rice, corn, whole-grain breads, bagels, and pastas, white potatoes, sweet potatoes, and squashes. To these central starches are added fresh or fresh-frozen fruits and vegetables. Some of the dishes you now enjoy fit or come close to our recommendations, like oatmeal or whole-grain cold cereals for breakfast; vegetable soups for lunch; and spaghetti or bean burritos for dinner. You will probably need to make some slight modifications in your choices, such as replacing skim milk with low-fat soy milk or rice milk, and leaving out the oil and the cheese on the lunch and dinner selections. Most people can add reasonable amounts of salt, sugar, and spices to their foods.

By nature, most people have a hard time moderating a bad habit and are better at simply quitting it cold. Most smokers, for example, just quit, they don't reduce their consumption from three packs to three cigarettes a day. Complete abstinence is, of course, essential for alcoholics and drug addicts. In matters of diet, incorporating a few ounces of the rich foods we were raised on, like the meats, makes temptation too great for most people. You have to face the tempters every time you open the refrigerator. Furthermore, some of your health problems may continue, because they are actually allergic responses to the proteins in the food, not to the fats. Even low-fat dairy products will continue to clog the sinuses, aggravate asthma, and provoke the painful inflammation of rheumatoid arthritis.

A Practical Way of Cooking

In an effort to provide interesting meals, promoters of some low-fat plans hire professional cooks and dietitians to help them—and it shows. Meal preparation becomes a day-long job; recipes call for professional skills and restaurant equipment. In other cases recipes are invented by professional dietitians who excel at determining the correct number of grams of fat, sodium, and cholesterol in your menu but have spent little time in the kitchen in front of a stove—and that, too, shows. The recipes in this book are designed with the home cook and (not incidentally) the person who enjoys good food in mind. They were developed by Mary McDougall and contributed by followers of the McDougall Program, none of whom is a dietician or professional chef. Mary is a mother and a homemaker, with many responsibilities besides food preparation. The job of feeding her family must be accomplished efficiently, and with enjoyable meals. Therefore, most of the recipes in this book are made from ingredients found in local supermarkets and take into account the individual preferences of all members in a family.

A Program Born Out of a Doctor's Frustration

Through four years of medical school, three years of postgraduate training in internal medicine, and my first four years of medical practice, I found the profession generally a disappointment. Like most doctors, I had dedicated my life to medicine because I wanted to help people. Unfortunately, the miracles encountered in my practice were few and far between. I could make a difference in some people's lives, especially those with acute (short-term) problems—cuts I could sew up, or minor infections I could treat with antibiotics. The majority of my patients, however, had chronic conditions, like obesity, heart disease, high blood pressure, diabetes, arthritis, indigestion, constipation, colitis, and multiple sclerosis. These problems resisted my efforts to correct them because I was relying primarily on bottles full of useless, and often harmful, pills dispensed to trusting patients.

Fortunately, I realized early in my career that the diseases from which most people suffer are caused by eating too much rich food. The problems caused by poor nutrition are compounded by physical inactivity, and sometimes by smoking and drinking. Exercise and other health habits had been addressed by many other physicians, but little had been said about the role that diet plays in the prevention and treatment of diseases. I began intensively researching this neglected aspect of medicine in 1976, while in a medical residency program in Hawaii. My goal was to find a dietary approach that would offer people the best chance of recovering from chronic illnesses. The way foods actually tasted was a distant second to this primary focus of my activity.

Mary's Creative Response

As I researched the medical literature, I began to understand the complete overhaul that needed to be made in the standard American diet—which was also my personal diet! And my health needed improvement as much as did that of any young man my age. I was a little overweight, always tired, and usually constipated, and suffered from some other medical complications as well.

So I put my ideas into practice, and our family gave up red meat for white. It was an easy decision, one made by many people in the 1970s. But when I discovered that chicken and fish contain as much cholesterol as do beef and pork, my scientific conscience forced a more significant change, all the way to vegetarianism. For a conservative member of the medical profession, that was a major change. Mary developed cheese- and egg-based dishes accordingly.

As I continued to study nutrition and disease, I discovered that America's most trusted food group—dairy products—was unhealthy as well. Cheese contains as much fat and cholesterol as steak. And milk, cheese, yogurt, cottage cheese, and ice cream can lead to a wide variety of diseases: food allergies, stomach distress, cancer, and heart attacks, to name only a few.

Even though I knew about the relationship between dairy products and such illnesses, and the fact that calcium was abundant in plants, and that milk was entirely unnecessary for the growth and health of my own children, I still had a hard time adjusting to this knowledge.

I remember standing in front of my opened refrigerator, bare of all dairy products, with my two young children, ages six and seven, beside me. "I must be an irresponsible parent," I worried. "What have I been doing? I haven't fed these kids any cow's milk!" That was "Elsie the Cow" talking to and through me. Years of watching television commercials had brainwashed me. All the scientific facts in the library still had trouble bulldozing through piles of that cow's propaganda. I can imagine how difficult it must be for other, less informed, parents, when they consider taking their kids off "Nature's Perfect Food." Even when they are confronted with the evidence that dairy products are making their children pudgy and sick, only determined parents will make the effort to change their family's diet. I know how hard it can be. When I told Mary that dairy products were nutritionally like "liquid meat" and that they would have to go, she almost said I had to go.

By the time my reading discovered the cancer-promoting and obesity-causing effects of vegetable oils, Mary was accustomed to my disrupting discoveries. She adjusted easily to using nonstick cookware and created methods for moistening foods without adding oil. By moving away from the "four basic food groups," we transformed ourselves and became healthier, trimmer followers of a diet based on familiar starches, like beans, corn, potatoes, rice, and pasta. (Because these foods are the central ingredients, we call this a *starch-based diet.*) Making the complete change took us a couple of years. Since the last elimination of oil, the McDougall Program has remained unchanged.

The Simple Rules

The most important concept to understand is that this is a starch-based diet. No longer think meat-, egg-, and dairy-based meals. When someone asked, "What's for dinner?" once upon a time you answered, "Chicken, roast beef, or pork chops." Now you'll tell them, "Spaghetti, potatoes, beans, or rice." To this offering of basics, you add fruits and vegetables. To serve satisfying meals, grains and starchy vegetables must be a substantial part of your meal plan. You and your family will be hungry all the time if you mistake the meal plan to consist mostly of salad, broccoli, and cauliflower, with half a grapefruit thrown in for dessert.

People love to eat these starches. Unfortunately, because of such popular misconceptions as "potatoes are fattening," and "you must eat meat for protein," and "milk is necessary for strong bones and teeth," Americans have avoided for too long the very foods the body needs for good health and an attractive appearance. Starches are the staple foods of people around the world who are trim for life and suffer from few of the diseases that threaten the health and happiness of Americans. Think of the slim Chinese or Japanese, who live primarily on rice. This is not a genetic peculiarity to Asians. When Asians move to this country and begin to eat a rich Western diet, they lose their immunity to obesity and the diseases of overindulgence.

In underdeveloped countries, like those in central Africa, populations are essentially free of heart disease, breast cancer, and colon cancer, but they may have other health problems related to poor sanitation and lack of good medical care. In technologically advanced societies, these basic problems have been corrected. But we have unwittingly introduced the diseases that affect wealthy people. You can have the best of both worlds by taking advantage of technology and development, in our fortunate country, but continuing to eat the kind of starch-based diet that has nourished most of the people who have ever lived on planet Earth.

Modifying Recipes: Ten Simple Steps

For successful modification of your diet, you must begin with a favorite recipe containing familiar ingredients, including cherished seasonings. Many of the recipes used in the McDougall books had their origins in other recipe books or were adapted from meals we enjoyed in restaurants. With a little alteration they have become McDougall recipes. What's missing from them are all the ingredients that can make you fat and sick. Recipe modification has the simple goal of eliminating animal products and vegetable oils, while emphasizing grains, vegetables, fruits, and flavorings. You will end up with leaner, cleaner, lighter versions of your favorite recipes, with colors, textures, aromas, and tastes much like those of the originals. To complete each new creation, you can give it a name that reminds you of the source—or, if you prefer, one that is entirely new.

To modify a recipe, follow these ten steps:

1. Choose an enjoyable recipe that already supplies plentiful amounts of starches, vegetables, or fruits.
2. Delete all animal products from the recipe, including red meat, poultry, fish, shellfish, eggs, cheese, milk, and other dairy products.
3. When necessary, make substitutions for animal products. Substitute low-fat soy milk or rice milk for cows' milk, and use Ener-G Egg Replacer as a binder instead of eggs.

4. Remove all obvious fats and vegetable oils from the recipe, including olive, corn, and safflower oils.
5. Replace oil, if necessary, with water, fruit juice, a fruit sauce, or other moisturizers (see page 70). Use natural vegetable "gels" to thicken and to mix salt, sugar, and spice with food (see page 72).
6. Substitute whole grains for refined products (brown rice instead of white rice, whole-wheat flour instead of white flour, etc.).
7. Add vegetables and legumes that have a "meaty" texture, like textured vegetable protein, seitan, beans, and mushrooms; and, for even richer texture, add soybean products, such as tofu.
8. Use salt and sugar sparingly when cooking; add more, if necessary, to the surface of the food at the table.
9. Adjust the recipe to taste with preferred spices.
10. Increase portion size in order to provide enough for healthy appetites. (Delightful discovery: You can eat more of this kind of food than you did on the American diet without the risk of gaining excess weight.)

Recipes Without Possibilities for Improvement

Creating a new and healthier recipe usually begins with one for a dish that is already based on starch, vegetable, or fruit components. Some recipes are impossible to modify, however, because doing so would mean eliminating practically all of the ingredients. For example, one of our readers sent Mary this recipe for Chocolate Coffee Cake and asked her to include it in this book.

ORIGINAL RECIPE

Chocolate Coffee Cake

⅓ cup flaked coconut
¼ cup chopped cashew nuts
¼ cup sugar
3 tablespoons butter or
margarine, melted
2 cups Bisquick

¼ cup sugar
1 egg
¾ cup milk
⅓ cup semisweet chocolate
pieces, melted

Nutritional Analysis

PERCENT OF CALORIES
Fat: 48%
Protein: 6%
Carbohydrate: 46% (mostly sugar)

Cholesterol: 176 mg per 1,000 calories
Dietary Fiber: 2 gm per 1,000 calories

This recipe is unmodifiable for our purposes, because it has none of the ingredients we consider health supporting and, therefore, no possibility as a McDougall-approved dish.

Reconsidering Oil

When I lecture I take a bottle of olive oil or corn oil with me. When someone asks, "How will I cook anything delicious if I can no longer use oil?" I respond by asking him to prove his love of oil by drinking some of it from this bottle I brought along. The audience invariably responds with a sickening moan and a few giggles. No one will drink from my bottle of oil. If they did so, their physical reaction would likely be retching, or even vomiting. Nor would anyone pour the oil over his or her head for me, if I asked. Consider the fact we take many steps to keep oil out of our surroundings. We use strong detergents on our dishes to remove it; if oil spills on the counter, we use a powerful "grease-cutting" cleaner. And the most unflattering description for a restaurant is "greasy spoon."

Embargo Oil for Health

Oil is commonly used by the food industries to increase the shelf life of their products and to add cheap calories. (Few of us need more of those.) More important, oil is the agent used to stick the salt to French fries and potato chips; oil holds sugar to doughnuts, and oil in salad dressings spreads spices over salad leaves. The secret to healthful and enjoyable cooking is to find new ways to include salt, sugar, and spices in your recipes—methods that do not use oil. Your health and appearance will benefit from it.*

The fat you eat will soon become the fat you wear.** The body usually disposes of the fat in your foods by storing it. The cost of transporting the fat from your fork to your body tissues is only 3 percent of the calories in the fat itself (compared to 30 percent of the calories needed to transform carbohydrates into stored fat). Dietary fat also detracts from your appearance by causing oily skin and hair and feeding the kinds of bacteria that cause acne.

Saturated fats from animal products plug up your arteries, in a disease process called *atherosclerosis,* which eventually leads to heart attacks and strokes. All fats promote the development of cancers of the breast, colon, prostate, and kidney. Vegetable oils are even stronger promoters of such cancers than are fats derived from animals. Fats are also involved in inflammatory arthritis (rheumatoid, lupus, psoriatic, and ankylosing spondylitis), multiple sclerosis, and gallbladder disease.

Removing fats and oils from your diet will make weight loss easy if you are overweight, and permanent too. Many disease processes can be relieved by improving your diet. Most remarkable are the reversal of atherosclerosis, elimination of angina (chest pains), correction of hormone imbalances, recovery from adult-type diabetes and inflammatory arthritis, prevention of attacks of multiple sclerosis and gallbladder inflammation, and resolution of oily skin and acne.

---

*A few of the Oriental recipes in this book offer the option of adding a sprinkle of sesame oil for flavoring. In no other way can you achieve sesame's distinct flavor. But use no more than ⅛ teaspoon.

**Fat* is the term commonly used to describe the saturated fats found in animal products, which are solid at room temperature. Oil is also pure fat, but the term usually describes unsaturated vegetable fats, which are fluid at room temperature.

Defatting Recipes

High-fat foods are easy to identify. Animal products, such as meat, poultry, milk and its byproducts, and eggs, are high in fat unless they have been specially processed. Most vegetable foods are low in fat. Notable exceptions are a few high-fat plant foods: coconuts, nuts (and nut butters), seeds (and seed spreads), avocados, olives, soybeans (and tofu and soy milk), and the oils processed from various seeds and grains, like sunflower seed and corn oil. These few exceptions are easily remembered.

Example: Defatting

ORIGINAL RECIPE	MARY'S MODIFICATION

Tabouli

1 cup bulgur
1 cup water
½ cup fresh lemon juice
⅔ cup olive oil
1 cup chopped fresh mint
1 cup chopped fresh parsley
½ cup finely diced red onion
2 teaspoons minced garlic
1 teaspoon freshly ground black pepper
½ teaspoon salt
4 tomatoes, chopped
1 large cucumber, chopped

Nutritional Analysis

PERCENT OF CALORIES
Fat: 60%
Protein: 4%
Carbohydrate: 35%

Cholesterol: 0 mg
Dietary Fiber: 6 gm per 1,000 calories

Tabouli

1 cup bulgur
2 cups boiling water
½ cup fresh lemon juice
½ cup chopped fresh mint
½ cup chopped fresh parsley
½ cup chopped scallion (green onion)
2 teaspoons minced garlic
1 teaspoon freshly ground black pepper
2 tomatoes, chopped
1 cup cooked garbanzo beans

Nutritional Analysis

PERCENT OF CALORIES
Fat: 6%
Protein: 14%
Carbohydrate: 80%

Cholesterol: 0 mg
Dietary Fiber: 10 gm per 1,000 calories

By leaving out the oil, in this case olive oil, you can cut the percentage of calories from fat from 60 to 6! Each 100 calories of the original salad has 6.9 grams of fat, while each 100 calories of Mary's version has only 0.8 grams of fat. Quite an important savings, especially since you now know that those grams of fat become your body fat.

Cholesterol: A Burden on Your Arteries

As highly efficient animals, human beings make all the cholesterol we need to build the walls of our living cells and to synthesize our sex hormones and vitamin D. We do not need any extra input from our diet; cholesterol is not a "necessary nutrient." Approximately 40 percent of the cholesterol we eat is absorbed from our intestines and flows into our bloodstream. The problem with this extra cholesterol is that we generally can't eliminate it at the rate we consume it. Dogs, cats, and other carnivores have livers with a seemingly unlimited capacity to excrete cholesterol. Scientists can feed large amounts of egg yolk to these animals, and their arteries will remain undamaged. It is almost impossible to induce atherosclerosis in dogs and cats.

Other animals, like human beings, have livers with limited capacities to excrete cholesterol. Atherosclerosis is easily produced in these animals when they are fed diets high in cholesterol. We might conclude from this that we were born with the wrong kind of livers—that we should have livers with the capacities of dogs' and cats'. Another possible conclusion is that we shouldn't eat like dogs and cats.

As millions of Americans have learned, cholesterol plays a key role in the processes that damage and weaken the arteries, thereby causing strokes and heart attacks. Cholesterol is also a major contributor to the formation of gallstones and to the provocation of other diseases. Approximately 20 percent of all Americans develop gallstones, and by retirement age the incidence has risen to 40 percent. Because of the serious burden placed on the body by cholesterol, it is important to avoid the culprit as much as possible, by choosing the right foods.

No Cholesterol in Plants

Cholesterol is found only in animal products, like beef, pork, chicken, turkey, fish, lobster, shrimp, milk, cheeses, and eggs. No cholesterol is found in any plant. To make a simple rule as to what foods you should and should not eat, draw an imaginary line between the animal and plant kingdoms. Avoid all animal foods, and choose healthful foods containing no cholesterol by eating only starches, vegetables, and fruits. Except for a few highly saturated plant fats, such as coconut oil, palm oil, cocoa butter, and manufactured shortenings and margarine, all plant foods help to lower cholesterol levels in the body. These few exceptions are easily remembered.

Example: Removing Cholesterol

ORIGINAL RECIPE	MARY'S MODIFICATION
## Turkey à la King	## Turkeyless à la King

ORIGINAL RECIPE

Turkey à la King

½ cup diced green pepper
One 6-ounce can sliced mushrooms, drained (reserve ¼ cup liquid)
½ cup butter or margarine
½ cup flour
1 teaspoon pepper
2 cups light cream
1¾ cups chicken broth
2 cups cubed turkey
One 4-ounce jar diced pimientos

MARY'S MODIFICATION

Turkeyless à la King

1 yellow onion, chopped
1 green pepper, chopped
½ pound mushrooms, cleaned and sliced
1 celery stalk, sliced
6 to 8 ears baby corn, cut in half
1 cup frozen peas
½ cup whole-wheat flour
3 cups soy or rice milk
One 4-ounce jar diced pimientos
1 to 2 teaspoons slivered fresh basil
⅛ teaspoon white pepper
2 tablespoons low-sodium soy sauce
1 tablespoon Worcestershire sauce
2 tablespoons cornstarch or arrowroot, mixed with ¼ cup cold water

Nutritional Analysis	*Nutritional Analysis*
PERCENT OF CALORIES Fat: 77% Protein: 14% Carbohydrate: 10%	PERCENT OF CALORIES Fat: 6% Protein: 15% Carbohydrate: 79%
Cholesterol: 302 mg per 1,000 calories Dietary Fiber: 2 gm per 1,000 calories	Cholesterol: 0 mg Dietary Fiber: 30 gm per 1,000 calories

By leaving the turkey, butter, and chicken broth out of the recipe, you can significantly lower the amounts of cholesterol and cholesterol-raising fats. This is quite important, given that one of the destinations of those 302 milligrams of cholesterol in the original recipe will be the arteries to your heart and brain (too soon leading to heart attacks and strokes in millions of people).

Animal Protein Is a Burden on Bones and Kidneys

To most Americans, eating healthier means choosing low-fat and low-cholesterol items. The food industry has responded by providing foods low in these two components. But when fat content is lowered in your diet, protein content is usually increased*— especially animal protein. Having been raised on incessant messages from the protein producers—the meat, egg, and dairy industries—many of us mistakenly regard protein as an "all American" nutrient. Research demonstrates otherwise. The medical truth is simply put: Excess proteins, especially the kinds present in animal products, place a serious burden on your health and promote many diseases.

We do need some protein for growth and repair of tissues, of

*Foods consist of three calorie-providing components—fat, protein, and carbohydrate. The total percent of each must add up to 100 percent of the calories in the food. When the percentage of fat is decreased the percent of protein and/or carbohydrate increases. If you're comparing the same amount of calories, then the absolute amount of either or both must increase also.

course, but the required amount is so small that it is virtually impossible to devise a diet that contains too little to meet the nutritional needs of adults and children. Not only is the absolute amount of needed protein always provided in starches and vegetables; the nutritional requirements for specific essential amino acids, the building blocks of proteins, are always met by these simple plant foods as well. Nature designed her foods to be complete—long before they reached the meddlesome attention of dietitians.

Excess protein is not stored; if it were, it would be stored as muscle, and we all would look like overdeveloped body builders. Excess protein is excreted from the body through the kidneys. In the process of excretion, the body loses its ability to retain calcium, and large amounts of this bone-building mineral are lost in the urine. The amount of calcium lost daily exceeds the amount of calcium absorbed from the intestine, resulting in a net loss, which must be made up from the calcium stores—the bones. The end result of years of calcium loss is osteoporosis, a disease of generalized bone loss that results in an increased risk of fractures, more common with age and in women. Excess minerals present in the urine can form kidney stones. Moreover, the excess protein found in the typical American diet also injures people's kidneys and liver. Reducing the quantity of protein consumed can be life saving for people already suffering from damage to these vital organs.

Moderating Proteins in Foods

Proteins from animal sources are more damaging than are proteins from plants. All starchy foods contain adequate, but not excessive, amounts of proteins, except for a few high-protein legumes—beans, peas, lentils, and their relatives. These few exceptions are easily remembered. In general, consumption of legumes should be limited to one cooked cupful a day. Some sensitive people may have to restrict their intake even further and take stricter measures to avoid excess protein. To make the rule simple, draw an imagined line between the animal and plant kingdoms, and eat more healthful foods offering the right amounts and kinds of proteins by selecting only starches, vegetables, and fruits.

Example: Improving Protein Amount and Kind

ORIGINAL RECIPE	MARY'S MODIFICATION

Old-fashioned Beef Stew

½ cup flour
1 teaspoon salt
¼ teaspoon pepper
2 pounds beef stew meat, cut into 1-inch pieces
2 tablespoons vegetable shortening
6 cups hot water
3 medium potatoes, pared and cut into 1-inch cubes
1 medium turnip, cut into 1-inch cubes
4 carrots, cut into 1-inch slices
1 green pepper, cut into strips
1 cup sliced celery (1-inch pieces)
1 medium onion, diced (about ½ cup)
1 tablespoon salt
2 beef bouillon cubes
1 bay leaf

Hearty Brown Stew

2 onions, sliced
2 celery stalks, sliced thickly
2 carrots, sliced thickly
3 potatoes, chunked
1 green pepper, cut into strips
½ pound mushrooms, quartered
2 to 3 cloves garlic
2 cups water
¼ cup low-sodium soy sauce
¼ cup tomato juice
½ tablespoon grated ginger
½ teaspoon dried marjoram
½ teaspoon dried thyme
½ teaspoon paprika
3 to 4 tablespoons cornstarch or arrowroot, mixed with ½ cup cold water

Nutritional Analysis	*Nutritional Analysis*
PERCENT OF CALORIES Fat: 35% Protein: 42% Carbohydrate: 23%	PERCENT OF CALORIES Fat: 3% Protein: 13% Carbohydrate: 84%
Cholesterol: 305 mg per 1,000 calories Dietary Fiber: 8 gm per 1,000 calories	Cholesterol: 0 mg Dietary Fiber: 24 gm per 1,000 calories

By leaving the beef out of the recipe, you can cut the percent of calories from protein from 42 to 13. This becomes even more important when you remember that animal protein is a much more serious burden on your health than is vegetable protein, robbing your bones of calcium and encouraging the formation of kidney stones.

Dairy Products Are the Last to Go

Dairy products are usually the last to go in the diet of people trying to be healthier. How could anything as wonderful as "mother's milk" be bad for you? you might ask. Mother's milk is certainly the ideal food for babies. Cow's milk is, inarguably, ideal for baby cows. But cow's milk is not fit for humans, adults or children. Milk is concentrated calories. After all, this is the primary food that enables a calf to grow from 100 pounds at birth to about 600 pounds in six months. Milk has a similar potential effect on the grown-up you. Because you can't grow any taller, however, you will grow larger in the only dimension you can—wider in all directions—with the aid of all those fat calories in milk.

In addition to promoting obesity, heart disease, and strokes, dairy fats also stimulate the growth of cancer of the breast, prostate, and colon. The proteins in dairy products are the leading cause of food allergy, and milk sugar, or lactose, which cannot be digested by most people in the world, causes diarrhea, stomach cramps, and intestinal gas. Dairy products are also deficient in several vitamins, dietary fiber, and iron. Iron-deficiency anemia is caused in young children, and (I believe) in most women, by a diet rich in dairy products.

Low-Fat Dairy Foods Still Promote Health Problems

Low-fat dairy products are an improvement over the high-fat varieties, of course, but fall far short of a satisfactory rating. When you remove the fat from a milk product, you increase the relative amounts of proteins and lactose. Consuming more protein increases one's likelihood of developing a food allergy and also promotes loss of calcium from the body, leading to osteoporosis. The low-fat varieties still cause lactose-induced bowel problems, as well as additional health problems resulting from fiber, mineral, and vitamin deficiencies.

Contamination

Dairy products often become contaminated with a variety of dangerous chemicals or infectious microbes. In one year, while I was living in Hawaii, milk was taken off the supermarket shelves on three separate occasions because of three different kinds of contamination. The first and most publicized disaster was contamination of milk with heptachlor from the chopped pineapple tops that are fed to dairy cows. Most chemicals are readily absorbed by animal fats because they are fat-soluble. Thus, as a result of this "bioconcentration," small quantities of pesticides, herbicides, and other chemical agents can reach dangerously high levels in the milk of cows.

The next sweep of milk from the shelves resulted from contamination with tuberculosis bacteria. Cow's milk is often polluted with other harmful microorganisms as well, such as those that cause salmonellosis, campylobacteriosis, and a number of viral infections. Some of the more sinister viruses found in cow's milk are bovine leukemia and bovine AIDS viruses. Over half of the dairy cows in this country are infected with these viruses. The leukemia viruses are transmittable under laboratory conditions to other species, like chimpanzees, who then develop leukemia. The incidence of human leukemia worldwide is in direct proportion to the amount of dairy products consumed. Think about these facts the next time you pour your child a glass of cold milk.

Residents of Hawaii were temporarily deprived of "Nature's Perfect Food" for the third time when too much penicillin got into the milk. Penicillin and many other antibiotics are used in feedlots and barnyards to keep the animals from becoming ill in those crowded conditions and to promote the growth of cows and the volume of milk they yield. The drug residues appear in the milk.

Avoid Dairy Products Completely

Foods from animals, including beef, poultry, dairy products, and eggs, share a similar potential for chemical contamination and for carrying disease-causing microorganisms. Most bacteria, fungi, and viruses that are adapted to infect plant hosts are so different from those infecting animals that they do not harm us. Because plant foods are low on the food chain and low in fat, the amounts of environmental contaminants present in their tissues are minimal. (Those sprayed on plant surfaces are another matter, of course.) Draw a line between the animal and plant kingdoms and choose more healthful foods with low levels of chemical contamination and almost no harmful microbes, by selecting only starches, vegetables, and fruits.

Example: Removing Dairy

ORIGINAL RECIPE	MARY'S MODIFICATION

Vichyssoise

1 large onion
¼ cup butter
4 medium potatoes,
  scrubbed and sliced
  thin
4 cups water
2 cups milk
½ pint heavy cream
1½ to 2 teaspoons salt
Freshly ground
  pepper
Freshly chopped
  scallions or chives

Vichyssoise

3 cups peeled and
  chunked potatoes
1½ cups chopped onion
½ cup sliced leek
5 cups water
⅛ teaspoon white
  pepper
1 tablespoon low-
  sodium soy sauce
1 cup low-fat soy milk
Freshly ground
  pepper to taste
Chopped scallions
  or chives for garnish

Nutritional Analysis

PERCENT OF CALORIES
Fat: 67%
Protein: 6%
Carbohydrate: 27% (mostly
  lactose)

Cholesterol: 249 mg per 1,000
  calories
Dietary Fiber: 7 gm per 1,000
  calories

Nutritional Analysis

PERCENT OF CALORIES
Fat: 3%
Protein: 10%
Carbohydrate: 86%

Cholesterol: 0 mg
Dietary Fiber: 15 gm per 1,000
  calories

By leaving the butter, milk, and cream out of this recipe, you can cut the percent of calories from fat from 67 to 3. You will also avoid ingesting milk protein, cholesterol, and lactose.

Good Health and Great Taste
at McDougall's

Once you understand the effect that the components in your foods have on your health and appearance, you'll realize that the only thing you'll give up by leaving out animal products and added oils is bad health—not a bit of delicious taste. Modifying recipes in favor of your health can be fun and challenging. Your old cookbooks and files are filled with recipes waiting to be rid of unhealthful ingredients. The recipes in this book will provide you with one new eating experience every day for almost a year.

CHAPTER 2

MAKING THE CHANGE

Change Can Be Bothersome . . .
or Exhilarating

Sometimes I think that for many people, far worse than the fear of public speaking, or for some few, the fear of dying from a dreaded disease, is the fear of changing their diet. They think, "Life will be worse—I'm not sure how, but I know it will be worse." "My social life will be ruined." "I'll never get to enjoy my favorite foods again." "The preparation of these new menus will make me a slave to the kitchen." Fear of making the change arises from an unwillingness to imagine how the new ways will bring them greater pleasure and comfort than did the old ways that had governed their eating habits for so many years.

The first step to making successful dietary changes is to admit that it *will* be troublesome, and you *will* have to devote considerable effort to make it happen. But isn't this exactly what happens with every new endeavor? If you don't make the commitment, you won't reap the benefits, whether you're learning to use a computer or how to program one of those newfangled VCRs.

*Packaged and canned products referred to in this section are listed on pages 42–69.

In preparing to make these changes you should list all the reasons why you want to improve the quality of your life by improving your diet. Motivations can be found in such areas as concern for your health and appearance, your religion, regard for ecology, and sympathy for the welfare of animals. Only you know which psychological buttons need to be pressed deep down inside you to persuade you to move from the place you are in now to a more healthful diet and a better lifestyle. Once you have made the decision to change, you can take the few steps needed to make the transition easier and more effective.

SAMPLE MOTIVATIONS

- I want to look better and feel better.
- I'm tired of the pain of indigestion.
- Daily laxatives must no longer be a part of my life.
- Frequent headaches must mean that something is wrong; they've got to stop.
- I'm too young to have painful arthritis.
- Breast cancer is a miserable and slow way to die; it's not for me.
- I fear that I won't live as long as my spouse will.
- Since childhood I've felt that something was wrong about eating the flesh of cows and lambs and piglets.
- America's hamburger habit is destroying our rain forests and the health of our planet.

All or Nothing?

Every positive experience you have with healthier eating is important in getting you to the day when you decide that you are worth the effort and are finally going to make the change. You may decide to start slowly by slipping in an occasional McDougall recipe along with your old favorites. There's nothing wrong with this approach, except that there will be a lot of heavy competition from those long-time favorite (and heavy) foods. Taking a "partway" approach can set you up to suffer slow withdrawal symptoms—and inevitable disappointment in your results. What is more, you won't gain the dramatic improvements in your health and appearance that the Program offers those who follow it strictly.

A complete change is actually easier and, of course, more effective. Most people, when they're given no other choice, adjust to the new tastes and methods of food preparation within three or four days. The McDougall Program helps you to do the best you can for yourself as quickly as possible.

You'll find two classes of recipes in this book: those that comply strictly with a starch-based diet and some that we consider "transitional treats." The latter call for high-fat plant products, such as tofu (54 percent fat), soy cheese (70 percent fat), soy milk (40 percent fat), nuts (80 percent fat), and olives (90 percent fat). These are rich foods meant only for special occasions and only for healthy people. And if you are not quite ready to eat according to the McDougall Program, you may find these recipes helpful when getting started. Trying these less-strict recipes will teach you two important things: first, that all the dishes are delicious; and second, that you are capable of learning to like these new preparations. The remainder of the recipes use ingredients that add 1 to 15 percent fat, resulting in a meal plan that is approximately 5 to 10 percent fat.

Challenges for Change

We have found that there are six basic challenges that people changing their diets encounter. They are an unaccustomed palate, resistance from friends and family, meal planning, shopping habits, cooking techniques, and seasoning foods.

Each of these topics will be discussed in the following pages.

Challenge #1:
The Unaccustomed Palate

SOLUTIONS

Go Exploring

You're up for the challenge; now you need to select a meal plan. This might seem like a formidable task. It will be simpler when you realize that your goal is to find a few favorites, no more than a dozen, to prepare and eat as often as you wish.

Most people's diets are simpler and more monotonous than they realize. All too often we eat the same thing for breakfast, whether our choice is bacon and eggs or oatmeal. Lunch is the same combination sandwich, day after day. For dinner we generally select from five or ten entrees. Every restaurant serves one favorite item that we choose frequently.

Join other people who will be following the program, explore the recipes in this and other McDougall books, and find about a dozen familiar dishes that you can repeat over and over again. In time you will modify this list by trying and adjusting to new recipes, which will soon become favorites.

Identify Familiar Dishes

Think about the textures and distinctive flavors of dishes you already like. Some meals in your present collection are close to being acceptable and need only minor modifications. For example, oatmeal is a popular breakfast. Instead of submerging it in milk, butter, or cream, try using low-fat soy milk or rice milk, fruit juice, or applesauce. If you want more flavor, sprinkle on a dash of cinnamon or a small amount of brown sugar. Try eating crisp hashbrown potatoes without the usual bath of grease. Instead, cook them without oil in a nonstick pan and serve them with catsup or barbecue sauce. Pancakes and waffles can be made from healthful ingredients and served with pure maple syrup.

Most soups are already vegetable-based. In making our kind of soup, simply leave out the usual starters of ham, chicken, or beef that contribute so much fat and cholesterol. Beans, corn, potatoes, and pasta will provide the more solid substance of your soups. Add salt, if it is tolerated, and appropriate spices to gain those appetizing flavors you like.

For evening meals you may already be enjoying dishes composed primarily of starches, vegetables, and fruits. Think about your favorite pasta and stew dishes. In preparing a rich red marinara sauce, you may only need to omit olive oil to transform it into a healthful and delicious topping for pasta.

Challenge #2: Resistance From Friends and Family

SOLUTIONS

Enroll Family and Friends

You yourself may be convinced that the McDougall Program is the best way known to science and medicine for you to eat, but your spouse, who has never been sick a day in his or her life, and wears the same size clothes as in high school, feels this message does not apply personally. Your children think your mind has been taken over by aliens from outer space. Heart disease and breast cancer worry them about as much as the possibility of a comet falling on them. Your friends whisper, "There goes Pat on another one of those get-healthy-quick schemes. It'll be something else next week."

Sure enough, changing your family's eating habits takes some work. You have to be creative in the kitchen, and you have to be patient with the doubting critics around the table. In most cases, you'll need no more than four months to "convert" the other members of your family. Your own success can help to persuade them, as they see you becoming more energetic and looking younger, and hear you telling them that you're feeling so much better.

Your concern about the welfare of close friends and family members may lead you to want to share this message with others. After changing your diet you will understand more about the causes and cures of disease than I knew years ago as a licensed physician before I discovered the importance of diet. You will have experienced firsthand the benefits that come from changing your diet, and should feel free to tell others about that happy experience if you want to.

Make Family-Style Meals

Take your family's preferences into consideration when planning meals. If they've always hated eggplant, don't make baked eggplant—they won't like it while on this program either. Always keep the importance of a starch-based diet in the forefront of your planning. Pasta dishes, soups, and breads are familiar and favorite foods, as are potatoes, in the form of hash browns, potato salad, and mashed potatoes; and beans, in the form of chili and baked beans.

If you can't get the full cooperation of every family member at the beginning, the best advice I can give is to prepare enough of your meal for everyone to share and then provide the others with a side dish of whatever they think they're missing—or, better yet, allow them to make it themselves. For example, if you serve spaghetti and a delectable oil-free marinara sauce (with their favorite spices in it), and you think they won't be happy without cheese and meatballs, then provide one or both as side dishes. When we have spaghetti in our home, an old pepper shaker with a big P on its side sits on the table. The children think this shaker holds Parmesan cheese. Actually, Mary fills it with soy "Parmesan cheese," and the kids don't know the difference.

Bean burritos can be served buffet-style. Start with corn and wheat tortillas. Set out small bowls of lettuce, tomatoes, onions, and sprouts. Different kinds of salsas should be placed at the end of the line. If your family is not yet satisfied with these offerings, because they're still longing for meats and salty dairy products, then put out a bowl of cow's cheese or soy cheese for them. You could also make a hamburger topping enhanced with meat seasonings. Better yet, these same seasonings can be mixed with textured vegetable protein (TVP; see the recipe in volume I of the McDougall cookbooks) for a "meaty" topping containing no cholesterol or animal fat. In the same considerate manner, offer a piece of chicken or fish as a side dish to a Mexican rice dinner. Be creative—even while you're indulging those holdouts still numbered among the unconverted.

Try cutting back on the mounds of meats and dairy foods you've been bringing to the table for too many years. Switch to soy bean–based alternatives. At the same time, increase the amount of starchy foods you serve. When eating "McDougall style," you may need to double the quantities you used to consume when eating a standard American diet in order to satisfy your appetite. That's okay; these are good calories.

Even at this early stage you have cut way back on the amounts of oil and cholesterol your family is consuming. Be quietly pleased with yourself: While the sum of your efforts may be appreciated only in the distant future, you're already winning an important battle on the calorie/cholesterol front.

Make Sure That Good Foods Are Available

The fastest way I know of to make the McDougall Program fail (just like all the other diets you've tried) is to give insufficient attention to buying good foodstuffs and then to preparing delicious meals from them. When the refrigerator and the cupboards are bare or, worse yet, filled with the old high-fat items that brought you to your alarming state of obesity and/or poor health, you're going to have a hard time fixing meals that please and ease.

Start by consulting other members of the family about dishes they would like to try. Have on hand assorted breads, bagels, pretzels, and crackers, all prepared with healthful ingredients. Leave a bowl of fresh fruit on a counter or table in a heavy-traffic area. Cut up fresh vegetables, and when not storing them in the refrigerator (in water, to maintain freshness), place them out to be eaten. Set prepared vegetable dips, spooned into plastic containers or still in their original packages, next to the vegetables. Cooked rice and baked potatoes, cold or hot, make quick snacks. Barbecue sauces, salad dressings, packaged soups, or leftover sauces and soups make easy toppings for cold cooked starches. Our refrigerator always holds a big bowl of cold boiled potatoes cleverly placed at eye level.

Challenge #3: Meal Planning

SOLUTIONS

Determine How Much Effort You're Willing to Make

When planning home-cooked meals for yourself and your family, begin by deciding how much time you are willing to spend in the kitchen. If you have been the kind of cook who burned a slice of animal flesh on two sides and called that dinner, then for you the healthy alternative is to microwave a potato or two and boil a bag of frozen vegetables. The nutrition derived from that offering will be excellent, and the flavor can be made pleasing by pouring on bottled oil-free salad dressings, salsas, spaghetti sauces, catsup, or barbecue sauces. (See the packaged-and-canned products list on pages 42–69.)

On the other hand, if you like to spend time in the kitchen, making meals from scratch, then a starch-based diet can be as simple or as elaborate as you wish. The recipes in our books contain detailed instructions for preparation of ingredients and accurate preparation and cooking times. The instructions are written simply and completely, so that even a novice cook should be successful on the first try.

Make a List

Begin by taking a few minutes to plan your menus for the week. Write down the ingredients you'll need to buy at the supermarket and the health-food store. A written list will save you time and money. Plan each meal around a starch food. Introduce variety by choosing different starches—you don't want to serve pasta three days in a row!

Serve Hearty Breakfasts

Traditional breakfast foods, like toast, cereals, pancakes, and waffles, made of whole grains, are already in line with the McDougall Program. Only a slight variation in the components of these dishes needs to be made. Many people can't imagine eating a breakfast cereal without milk or cream. The simple solution for hot cereal is to make it with a little extra water and top the mix with a sweetener, like brown sugar (if your health allows) or applesauce. If you need to pour something white on a hot or cold cereal, use rice milk or low-fat soy milk (purchased in a store; or try the recipe for these "milks" on pages 90 and 91). I enjoy fruit juice on my cold cereal. It provides not only moisture but also the flavor of the fruit and some degree of sweetness. Many cereal manufacturers already add fruits to cereals, taking advantage of this pleasurable combination of tastes.

Hash-brown potatoes are a favorite in our home. They can be made from scratch or purchased frozen in boxes and bags. Pour the desired amount of potatoes from the bag into a nonstick frying pan or wok, and cook for 20 to 25 minutes over medium heat, stirring occasionally. Compressed square patties of shredded potatoes sold in boxes of four to eight are my favorite. These become brown on a nonstick griddle after about 10 minutes per side at medium heat with a gas stove. (An electric stove takes a little longer.)

We add variety to our breakfasts of hash-brown potatoes at the dining table. Our daughter, younger son, and Mary top their potatoes with three different brands of bottled mild salsa. Our older son uses catsup. I use a mixture of Lea & Perrins Sauce and Bull's Eye Barbecue Sauce (quite a tangy taste). The possibilities for toppings are endless: try oil-free salad dressings, horseradish, Tabasco, Worcestershire sauce, packaged (or leftover) soup, spaghetti sauce, or any other favorite topping made with the right ingredients (no oils, no animal products, and only minimal amounts of salt, sugar, and additives unless you can't tolerate these)

A simple and fast breakfast can be a bagel, a piece of toast, or a rice cake, plain or topped with sugar-free jam. Recipes for more complicated breakfasts can be found in this book. There's nothing sacred about what you eat for breakfast. I'm sure you've had left-over pizza or a burrito for breakfast in the past. You can do the same with healthy foods and have for breakfast things that are customarily reserved for lunch or dinner. The first meal of the day in Asian countries is often the same as the middle and the last meal: rice and vegetables.

Hot drinks for breakfast should be noncaffeinated (because caffeine has adverse health effects for many people such as anxiety and rapid, irregular heartbeat). Try cereal beverages like Postum, Caffix, and Pero. Herb teas are satisfying selections. Some people enjoy hot water with lemon juice. Fruit juices are excellent cold drinks, although some people can't tolerate them well because of indigestion caused by acidity.

Provide a Tasty Lunch

Lunch is usually a hurried affair, because it falls during the working part of our day. Leftovers make easy lunches as they are. Bean or grain dishes, and soups left to thicken as they cool, make great sandwich stuffings. For variety, add lettuce, sprouts, sliced tomatoes, and onions, along with dashes of a bottled sauce (Tabasco, barbecue sauce, or steak sauce), or of an oil-free salad dressing, or one of the many mustards available.

Do you usually manage to fill your pita-bread pocket too full? If so, separate the pita bread in half by cutting around its edge, leaving two flat circles. Layer the foods you want over one half and cover with the other; eat the combination like a sandwich or with a fork and knife. You can also spread leftovers on your circles of pita bread and add garnishes and sauces; then roll up the filled circle like a burrito.

Some instant dry soups packaged in paper containers make excellent lunches. Just add hot water and wait a couple of minutes for lunch to be ready. Instant soups come in many varieties. (See the packaged-and-canned products list on pages 42–69.)

Potatoes are another great foundation for lunches. Bake, boil, or microwave them. Cut crosswise in half, split lengthwise down the middle, or mash the white of the potato, or the white and skin, before adding a topping. Instant dry packaged soups can be made with half the recommended volume of hot water and then poured over a cooked potato, providing a substantial covering with spicy flavors. Also try oil-free salad dressings, salsas, barbecue sauces, catsup, steak sauces, horseradish, Tabasco, Worcestershire sauce, spaghetti sauce, or any other favorite sauce (oil- and animal product-free, of course) on your potatoes.

If you pack a lunch for work or school, use covered plastic containers. Carry cooked potatoes in a sealed plastic bag. Soups and other liquids can be stored hot or cold in a Thermos. Fresh tap water, bottled mineral water, juices, and bags of herb teas are convenient beverages for packed lunches.

Make a Satisfying Dinner

Your dinners will be planned around starches, with the addition of fresh or frozen vegetables and fruits, mixed with your favorite seasonings. Your first goal is to decide on a few selections that will please everyone who will share the meals.

Keep It Simple

When we first started eating this way more than fifteen years ago, Mary would make three or four different dishes for a meal, in an effort to imitate the American style of serving a main dish, two or three side dishes, and a dessert. But she soon learned that too much variety makes for too much work. In the old days, for most people, meals were simple: porridge for breakfast, soup for lunch, and a stew for dinner. You, too, should plan your meals around a single dish, perhaps supplementing it with a salad or vegetable side dish. Think of pasta with a topping, or rice covered with a sauce, or just plain soup and wholesome bread.

Make Quantities

You may be concerned about the large yields of some of Mary's recipes if you are cooking for only one or two "small eaters." But we suggest that you still make at least the full quantity called for in a recipe and refrigerate or freeze the leftover portions. This will save you preparation time later, as well as money, and will enable you to have something tasty on hand for a future meal. All of these foods freeze well, except those made with arrowroot or cornstarch, which become sort of lumpy when frozen. If you plan to freeze foods containing these thickeners, you should separate and freeze the surplus amounts without adding the cornstarch or arrowroot. Add the arrowroot or cornstarch to the separated portions later, when you heat them.

Make an extra effort to have on hand portions of frozen beans and rice. This will cut down on preparation time for recipes that use these slow-cooking foods.

Challenge #4: Shopping Habits

SOLUTIONS

Find a Good Supermarket and Natural-Food Store

With the list you've made for the week's menus, start shopping at your local supermarket. Pick a market that supplies good fresh fruits and vegetables. Many of the upscale markets have health-food and specialty sections, where some of the unusual ingredients can be found.

We shop in a natural-foods store about once a month, stocking up on the items we cannot find in a supermarket. (A natural-foods store puts emphasis on *foods*, not on vitamin and mineral supplements and protein powders.)

Read Labels

The key to effective shopping is careful reading of labels. Ingredients are supposed to be listed in descending order of amounts. Manufacturers can deceive you with the present food labels, however. For example, simple sugars, like sucrose, corn syrup, fructose, and fruit concentrate, might be listed individually, so that *sugar* isn't the first ingredient on the list.

Manufacturers have found clever ways of hiding fats in ingredient lists by calling them *monoglycerides* or *diglycerides*. You might recognize *triglyceride* as being a complex fat but would probably overlook the mono- and di- forms, mistaking them for additives, unrelated to fats. The chemical difference among these three is the number of chains of fatty acids attached to the backbone molecule (glycerol): 1 (mono), 2 (di), or 3 (tri). Lecithin is another fat you may not recognize as such. Most lecithin is made from soybeans and is no more effective at lowering cholesterol in the blood than is any other vegetable oil.

You want to avoid fat as much as possible. Look for oils on product labels and avoid these products. (You will often find 1 gram of fat listed on the label of an apparently no-added-fat product. This 1 gram represents the total amount of fats in naturally low-fat vegetable foods.)

The FDA is in the process of improving labels to help you better judge the contents of a package. When you're buying packaged foods, be sure to read the ingredient labels carefully. And then read them again periodically, to catch changes in manufacturing practices and advertising ploys.

FIGURING PERCENT OF CALORIES

A little simple math will help you determine how much fat, protein, and carbohydrate are in a labeled food or packaged product.

Example product: Oatmeal
Total calories 100
Fat 2g
Protein 5g
Carbohydrate 18g

Percent fat is calculated by multiplying the number of grams of fat by *9 calories per gram*, dividing the answer (the number of calories of fat) by the total calories, then multiplying by 100 percent. Your daily goal is less than 10 percent fat.

2 g fat × 9 calories/gram = 18 calories ÷ 100 calories × 100% = 18% fat

Percent protein is calculated by multiplying the number of grams of protein by *4 calories per gram*, dividing the answer (the number of calories of protein) by the total calories, then multiplying by 100 percent. Your daily goal is 8 to 15 percent protein.

5 g protein × 4 calories/gram = 20 calories ÷ 100 calories × 100% = 20% protein

Percent carbohydrate is calculated by multiplying grams of carbohydrate by *4 calories per gram*, dividing the answer (the number of calories of carbohydrate) by the total calories, then multiplying by 100 percent. Your daily goal is 75 to 87 percent carbohydrate.

18 g carbohydrate × 4 calories/g = 72 ÷ 100 × 100% = 72% carbohydrate

Please note because the grams are rounded off to the nearest whole number on the package label the calculated percentages will rarely add up to 100% as they should.

Order Supplies by Mail

People living in rural areas will be unable to find some of the specialty items called for in our recipes in their local grocery stores. Mail-order houses can solve this problem. You can save 30 to 50 percent on your purchases by buying in bulk from some of these places. If the minimum bulk order (generally $200 to $500) is too much for you to manage, then team up with friends on an order. (See the Appendix for a list of mail-order stores.)

Choose Canned and Packaged Products Carefully

Acceptable canned and packaged products are those free of added oils and animal products. Many, however, do contain salt, sugars, spices, and additives that some people cannot tolerate. Read the labels carefully before deciding to buy. Manufacturers will sometimes change the ingredients in a product, so check labels periodically.

McDougall-Okayed Packaged and Canned Products

MANUFACTURER/DISTRIBUTOR   VARIETY

Cold Cereals

These cereals are made with whole grains, are low in salt, sugar, and additives, and contain no added fats or oils.

Nabisco	Shredded Wheat
Post	Grape-Nuts
Nature's Path Foods	Manna (Millet Rice Flakes, Multi-Grain Flakes), Fiber O's Corn Flakes
Kölln	Oat Bran Crunch
Health Valley Foods	100% Natural Bran Cereal Oat Bran Flakes Oat Bran O's Blue Corn Flakes Stone Wheat Flakes Raisin Bran Fruit Lites Fiber 7 Flakes
U.S. Mills	Uncle Sam (Erewhon) Crispy Brown Rice (Erewhon) Raisin Bran (Erewhon) Wheat Flakes Skinner's Raisin Bran Skinner's Low-Sodium Raisin Bran
Perky Foods	Crispy Brown Rice Nutty Rice
Barbara's Bakery	Brown Rice Crisps Breakfast O's Breakfast Biscuits Raisin Bran

MANUFACTURER/DISTRIBUTOR   VARIETY

Cold Cereals (continued)

Kellogg Co.   Nutri-Grain (Corn, Wheat, Nug-
                                          gets, etc.)

Weetabix Co.   Grainfields (Wheat Flakes, Raisin
                                          Bran, Corn Flakes)
                                        Wheetabix Whole Wheat Cereal

Arrowhead Mills   Wheat Flakes
                                        Bran Flakes
                                        Oat Bran Flakes
                                        Corn Flakes
                                        Puffed Wheat
                                        Puffed Rice
                                        Puffed Millet
                                        Puffed Corn

New Morning   Fruit-e-O's
                                        Super Bran
                                        Oatios

Trader Joe's   Fat-Free Granola—Apple Straw-
                                          berry

Alvarado St. Bakery   Organic Granola

Health Valley   Fat-Free Granola

Breadshop   Health Crunch

Hot Cereals

These cereals are made with whole grains, are low in salt, sugar, and
additives, and contain no added fats or oils.

Mercantile Food Co.   American Prairie Organic Hot
                                          Cereals

Quaker Oats Co.   Quaker Oats
                                        Quick Quaker Oats

MANUFACTURER/DISTRIBUTOR	VARIETY

Hot Cereals (continued)

U.S. Mills (Erewhon)

Instant Oat Meal
Barley Plus
Brown Rice Cream

Stone-Buhr Milling

Hot Apple Granola
7-Grain Cereal

Golden Temple Bakery

Oat Bran

Barbara's Bakery

14 Grains

Kashi Company

Kashi (some sesame seeds)

Arrowhead Mills

Bear Mush
Cracked Wheat
7 Grain
Oat Bran
Instant Oatmeal

Maple Leaf Mills

Red River Cereal (Original, Creamy Wheat, and Bran)

Pritikin Systems

Hearty Hot Cereal (Apple Raisin Spice)

Lundberg Family Farms

Rice Cereal

Frozen Potatoes

Frozen potatoes have no added fats, oils, or salt. Most have sugar (dextrose) and a preservative added (Mr. Dell's are pure potatoes.)

Ore-Ida Foods

Hash Browns
Potatoes O'Brien

Bel-air

Hash Browns

Mr. Dell Foods

Hash Browns

J.R. Simplot Co.

Okray's Hash Brown Potato Patties

MANUFACTURER/DISTRIBUTOR   VARIETY

Popcorn

These contain unprocessed popcorn only, with no added ingredients. You can pop any natural popcorn yourself in an air popper or in the microwave.

H.J. Heinz Co.	Weight Watchers Microwave Popcorn
Nature's Best	Nature's Cuisine (natural popcorn)
Energy Food Factory	Poprice
Lapidus Popcorn Co.	Lite-Corn
Specialty Grain Co.	Pop-Lite Microwave Popcorn
Country Grown Foods	Gourmet Popcorn

Rice Cakes

These products are made of rice with other whole grains and seasonings, and have no added fats or oils. Some have added salt.

Quaker Oats Co.	Rice Cakes (lightly salted) Corn Cakes Caramel Corn Cakes
H.J. Heinz Co.	Chico San (Millet, Buckwheat, and more)
Hollywood Health Foods	Mini Rice Cakes (Teriyaki, Apple Cinnamon)
Pacific Rice Prod.	Mini Crispys (Apple Spice, Raisin 'N' Spice, Italian Spice, Natural Sodium Free)
Westbrae Natural Foods	Teriyaki Rice Cakes
Lundberg Family Farms	Rice Cakes (Wild Rice, Wehani, Brown Rice, Mochi Sweet)

MANUFACTURER/DISTRIBUTOR   VARIETY

Rice Cakes (continued)

Lundberg Family Farms	Brown Rice Chewies
	Brown Rice Crunchies
	Organic Brown Rice
	Mini Rice Cakes
Glenn Foods	Brown Rice Treat

Crackers

These crackers are made of rice, wheat, rye, and other whole grains with seasonings, and have no added fats or oils. Some have added salt.

San-J International	Brown Rice Crackers
Westbrae Natural Foods	Brown Rice Wafers
Ralston Purina Co.	Natural Ry-Krisp
Edward & Sons Trading Co.	Baked Brown Rice Snaps
Parco Foods	(Hol-Grain) Brown Rice Lite Snack Thins
	Whole Wheat Lite Snack Thins
O. Kavli A/S	Kavli Norwegian Crispbread
Barbara's Bakery	Crackle Snax
	Lightbread
Sandoz Nutrition Corp.	Wasa Crispbread (Lite Rye, Hearty Rye)
H.J. Heinz Co.	Weight Watchers Crispbread (Harvest Rice)
Shaffer, Clarke & Co.	Finn Crisp

MANUFACTURER/DISTRIBUTOR   VARIETY

Crackers (continued)

Lifestream Natural Foods   Wheat & Rye Krispbread

Nabisco   Fat Free Premium Crackers

Baja Bakery   Rice & Bean Tortilla Bites

Edward & Sons Trading Co.   Brown Rice Sembei

Snack Cracks   Organic Rice Crackers (tamari,
                                  lightly salted)

Soken Products   Sesame Wheels (brown rice)

Pretzels

These contain no added fats or oils. Most are high in salt, and are made with refined flours.

Laura Scudder's   Mini-Twist Pretzels
                                  Pretzel Sticks
                                  Bavarian Pretzels

Anderson Bakery Co.   Oat Bran Pretzels

Snyder's of Hanover   Sourdough Hard Pretzels (salted
                                  and unsalted)

Granny Goose Foods   Stick Pretzels 100% Natural
                                  Bavarian Pretzels (salted
                                  and unsalted)

J & J Snack foods   Super Pretzels (frozen)

Barbara's Bakery   Barbara's Whole Wheat Bavarian
                                  Pretzels

MANUFACTURER/DISTRIBUTOR   VARIETY

Chips

H.J. Heinz Co.   Weight Watchers Apple Chips

Guiltless Gourmet   Guiltless Gourmet No Oil Tortilla
                                        Chips

Barbara's Bakery   Basically Baked Organic Tortilla
                                        Chips

Trader Joe's   Baked Tortilla Chips

El Galindo Mexican Foods   Oil-Free Salted Baked Tortilla
                                        Chips
                                        Oil-Free Blue Corn Baked Tortilla
                                        Chips

Synergy Systems Corp.   Childers Natural Potato Chips

Breads

These breads are baked with whole wheat, sprouted wheat, rye, or
other whole-grain flours, and have no added oil or dairy products,
such as whey.

Cedarlane Foods   Whole Wheat Lavash Bread

Lifestream Natural Foods   Essene Bread

Nature's Path Foods   Manna Bread

Grainaissance   Mochi (Plain, Raisin Cinnamon,
                                        Mugwort, Organic)

International Baking Co.   Mr. Pita

Garden of Eatin'   Bible Bread (regular and salt-free)
                                        Thin-Thin Bread

Breads For Life   Sprouted 7-Grain Bread
                                        Sprouted Wheat with Raisin
                                        Sprouted Rye Bread

MANUFACTURER/DISTRIBUTOR	VARIETY

Breads (continued)

Interstate Brands	Pritikin Bread (Rye, Whole Wheat, Multi-Grain)
French Meadow Bakery	French Meadow Brown Rice Bread
New England Foods Co.	Whole Wheat Milldam Pouch Bread
Food For Life	Sprouted Grain Breads
Great Harvest Bread Co.	Great Harvest Bakery (Honey Wheat) 9-Grain Rye Onion Dill Country Whole Wheat
Brother Juniper's Bakery	Oil-Free Breads (Cajun Three Pepper, Oreganato, Whole Wheat)
Alvarado St. Bakery	Oil-Free Breads and Buns
Siljans Knacke	Swedish Dark Rye Crispbread
Norganic Foods Co.	Katenbrot (Rye Bread)
Ryvita	Crisp Breads
Burns & Ricker	Crispini
Nokomis Farms	Country Loaf (Sourdough)
Snack Cracks	Pizza Crust (Organic Brown Rice)
Oasis Breads	Creative Crust Dinner Shells

Breads (continued)

Trader Joe's   Force Primeval Bars (Raisin Wal-
                                     nut Apple Bars)
                                  Raisin Rolls Choyce

Health Valley   Fat Free Muffins

Soups

These soups have no meat, dairy, or added fats and oils. Many are
high in salt.

Dry Packaged
Nile Spice Foods   Cous-Cous (Tomato Minestrone,
                                     Lentil Curry, Lentil, Black
                                     Bean, Split Pea)
                                  Chili 'n' Beans

Westbrae Natural Foods   Ramen (Whole Wheat, Onion,
                                     Curry, Carrot, Miso, Seaweed,
                                     5 Spice, Spinach, Mushroom,
                                     Buckwheat, Savory Szechuan,
                                     Oriental Vegetable, Golden
                                     Chinese)
                                  Instant Miso Soup (Mellow
                                     White, Hearty Red)
                                  Noodles Anytime (Country Style)

Sokensha Co.   Soken Ramen

Eden Foods   Buckwheat Ramen
                                  Whole Wheat Ramen

Wil-Pak Foods   Taste Adventure Soups (Black
                                     Bean, Curry Lentil, Split Pea,
                                     Red Bean)

Fantastic Foods   Fantastic Soups (Leapin Lentils
                                     Over Couscous, Fantastic
                                     Rockin' ABC's, Fantastic
                                     Jumpin' Black Beans,

MANUFACTURER/DISTRIBUTOR   VARIETY

Soups (continued)

	Fantastic Splittin' Peas, Pinto Beans and Rice Mexicana)
The Spice Hunter	Kasba Curry with Rice Bran Mediterranean Minestrone
Canned Health Valley	Fat-Free Soups (5 Bean Vegetable & Country Corn and Vegetable, plus others)
Real Fresh	Andersen's Soup (Split Pea)
Hain Pure Food Co.	Fat-Free Soup (Vegetarian Split Pea, Vegetarian Veggie Broth)
Mercantile Food Co.	American Prairie Vegetable Bean Soup
Trader Joe's	Mostly Unsplit Pea Soup

Burger Mixes/Meat Substitutes

These mixes contain no added fats, oils, or dairy products. Most tell you to fry in oil—*don't.* Cook on a nonstick griddle.

Fantastic Foods	Fantastic Falafil Nature's Burger (Barbecue Flavor)
Lima	Seitan (a wheat-derived meat substitute)
Santa Fe Organics	Hickory Smoked Seitan and others
Arrowhead Mills	Seitan Quick Mix

Burger Mixes/Meat Substitutes (continued)

Vegetarian Health Society	Vegetarian Hamburger Bits
	Vegetarian Beef Chunks
Worthington Foods	GranBurger
Lightlife Foods	Smart Dogs (meatless hot dogs)
Fearn Natural Foods	Breakfast Patty Mix

Pastas

These pastas are made without eggs or added oils or fat. Most are made of flour and water only and are low in sodium.

Health Valley Foods	Spaghetti Pasta (Spinach, Whole Wheat, Amaranth, etc.)
Westbrae Natural Foods	Spaghetti Pasta (Spinach, Whole Wheat)
	Lasagna Noodles (Spinach, Whole Wheat)
	Whole Wheat Somen, Udon, Soba
DeBole's Nutritional Foods	Curly Lasagna
	Elbows
	Spaghetti
	Corn Pasta (Wheat-free)
Quinoa Corp.	Quinoa Spaghetti (Wheat-free)
Golden Grain Macaroni Co.	Spaghetti
	Macaroni
	Rotini
	Lasagna
	Manicotti
A. Zerega's Sons	Antoine's Pasta (Fusilli Tri Colori)
Eden Foods	Udon (Japanese Noodles)

MANUFACTURER/DISTRIBUTOR	VARIETY

Pastas (continued)

Eden Foods	Soba (buckwheat) Japanese Rice Pasta Eden Vegetable Pastas (organic)
Nanka Seimen Co.	Chow Mein Udon
Sokensha Co.	Soken Jinenjo Noodles
Health Foods	MI-del (Spaghetti, Macaroni, Alphabets)
Best Foods, CPC Int.	Muellers (Twist, Spaghetti, Linguine)
Borden	Creamette (Spaghetti, Fettuccini, Rotini, Shells)
Reese Finer Foods	Da Vinci Pasta
Ferrara Foods	Gnocchi with Potato
Ronzoni Foods Corp	Radiatore-79 Linguine Fusilli Rotelle Spaghetti
Pastariso Products	Brown Rice Pasta (wheat free)
Food For Life Baking Co.	Wheat-Free Rice Elbows
Bertagni	Gnocchi di Palate
Amway Corp.	Microwave Pasta Ribbons

MANUFACTURER/DISTRIBUTOR   VARIETY

Pastas (continued)

Mrs. Leeper's Inc.   Michelle's Natural 2 Minute
                           Pasta (Vegetable Medley Angel
                           Hair)

Dry Packaged Grains and Pastas

These contain whole grains only, with no added fats or oils.

Health Valley Foods   Oat Bran Pasta with Sauce
                            (Fettucini Marinara, Fettucini
                            Primavera)

Quinoa Corp.   Quinoa

Continental Mills   ala—cracked wheat bulgur

Lundberg Family Farms   Rizcous (grain mixture—don't
                              follow cooking directions—
                              omit butter and olive oil)

Fantastic Foods   Brown Basmati Rice
                        Whole-Wheat Couscous

Arrowhead Mills   Wholegrain Teff
                        Wheat-Free Oatbran Muffin Mix
                        Griddle Lite Pancake & Baking
                          Mix
                        Quick Brown Rice (Spanish Style,
                          Vegetable Herb, and Wild Rice
                          & Herbs)

Pritikin Systems   Mexican Dinner Mix
                         Brown Rice Pilaf

Near East Food Prod.   Spanish Rice
                             Wheat Pilaf
                             Taboule
                             Lentil Pilaf Mix

Sahara Natural Foods   Casbah (Wheat Pilaf, Spanish
                             Pilaf, Whole-Wheat Couscous)

MANUFACTURER/DISTRIBUTOR   VARIETY

Dry Packaged Grains and Pastas (continued)

Nile Spice Foods	Whole Wheat Couscous Couscous Salad Mix Rozdali
Wil-Pak Foods	Taste Adventure (Black Bean Flakes and Pinto Bean Flakes)
J.A. Sharwood & Co.	Sharwood's India Pilau Rice
Texmati Rice	Basmati Brown Rice
Tipiak	Couscous
Liberty Imports	Instant Polenta
Jerusalem Natural Foods	Jerusalem Tab-ooleh
Aurora Import & Dist.	Polenta
Berhanu International Ltd.	Authentic Olde World—Lentils Divine

Bean and Vegetable Dishes (frozen or refrigerated)

Tumaro's	Black Bean Enchiladas
Amy's Kitchen	Amy's Organic Mexican Tamale Pie
United Foods	Pictsweet Express Microwaveable Vegetables
Bird's Eye, General Foods	Country Style Rice (microwave)

Salad Dressings

These contain no dairy products (whey, buttermilk, etc.), no fats or oils. (Many state clearly *No oil.*) Should also say low-sodium.

MANUFACTURER/DISTRIBUTOR   VARIETY

Salad Dressings (continued)

Pritikin Systems	No-oil Dressing (Ranch, Tomato, Italian, Russian, Creamy Italian, etc.)
WM Reily & Co.	Herb Magic (All No-oil—Vinaigrette, Italian, Gypsy, Zesty Tomato, Creamy Cucumber)
American Health Products	El Molino Herbal Secrets (All No-oil—Herbs & Spices, etc.)
Kraft	Oil Free Italian (high salt)
H.J. Heinz Co.	Weight Watchers Dressing (Tomato Vinaigrette, French)
Cook's Classics	Cook's Classic Oil-Free Dressings (Italian Gusto, Country French, Garlic Gusto, Dijon, Dill)
St. Mary Glacier	St. Mary's Oil Free Salad Dressing—many flavors
Trader Joe's	No-Oil Dill & Garlic Dressing, Italian
Sweet Adelaide Enterprises	Paula's No-Oil Dressing
Nature's Harvest	Oil-Free Vinaigrette, Oil-Free Herbal Splendor
Nakano USA	Seasoned Rice Vinegar
Uncle Grant's Foods	Uncle Grant's Salute—Honey Mustard Tarragon Dressing
S & W Fine Foods	Vintage Lites Oil-Free Dressing

MANUFACTURER/DISTRIBUTOR   VARIETY

Salad Dressings (continued)

Tres Classique	Grand Garlic Tomato & Herb French Dressing
The Mayhaw Tree	Vidalia Onion Vinegar

Spaghetti Sauce

These contain no meat, dairy products, or added oils or fats.

Pure & Simple	Johnson's Spaghetti sauce
Trader Joe's	Trader Giotto's Italian Garden Fresh Vegetable Spaghetti Sauce
Westbrae Natural Foods	Ci' Bella Pasta Sauce (no salt, no oil)
H.J. Heinz Co.	Weight Watchers Spaghetti Sauce with Mushrooms
Campbell Soup Co.	Healthy Request Marinara Sauce
S & W Fine Foods	Pasta Sauce
Pritikin Systems	Spaghetti Sauce (Original, Chunky Garden Style)
Beatrice/Hunt-Wesson	Healthy Choice Spaghetti Sauce
Nature's Harvest	Rocket Pesto
Tree of Life	Fat-Free Pasta Sauce
Sonoma Gourmet	Tomato Caper Herb Sauce

Soy Sauces

These contain no MSG (monosodium glutamate). They are all high in sodium, but some are sodium reduced.

MANUFACTURER/DISTRIBUTOR   VARIETY

Soy Sauces

Kikkoman Foods	Kikkoman Lite Soy Sauce
Westbrae Natural Foods	Mild Soy Sauce
San-J International	Tamari Wheat Free Soy Sauce
Live Food Products	Bragg Liquid Aminos
Edward & Sons Trading Co.	Ginger Tamari

Other Sauces

These sauces contain no oils, fats, or MSG. Many have salt and preservatives. Some are very spicy.

Trader Joe's	Zucchini Relish
New Morning	Corn Relish
Nabisco Brands	A1 Steak Sauce
Lea & Perrins	Lea & Perrins Steak Sauce HP Steak Sauce
Oak Hill Farms	Vidalia Onion Steak Sauce Three Pepper Lemon Hot Sauce
Reese Finer Foods	Old English Tavern Sauce
San-J International	Teriyaki Sauce
St. Giles Foods Ltd.	Matured Worcestershire Sauce
McIlhenny Co.	Tabasco
Gourmet Foods	Cajun Sunshine
Durkee-French Foods	Red Hot Sauce

MANUFACTURER/DISTRIBUTOR   VARIETY

Other Sauces (continued)

Baumer Foods	Crystal Hot Sauce
B.F. Trappey's Sons	Red Devil Louisiana Hot Sauce
J. Sosnick & Son	Kosher Horseradish
Reese Finer Foods	Prepared Horseradish
Aylas Organics	Szechwan, Cajun, Curry Sauce
Edward & Sons Trading Co.	Stir Krazy Vegetarian Worcester-shire Sauce

Salsas

These contain vegetable ingredients only, with no oils. Some have preservatives. Many have sugar and/or salt added.

Hain Pure Food Co.	Salsa
Pet	Old El Paso Salsa
Tree of Life	Salsa
Nabisco Brands	Ortega Green Chile Salsa
Pace Foods	Picante Sauce
La Victoria Foods	Chili Dip Salsa Jalapeña, etc.
Ventre Packing Co.	Enrico's Salsa
Guiltless Gourmet	Picante Sauce
Pritikin Systems	Salsa
Trader Joe's	Salsa Authentica Salsa Verde
Nature's Harvest	Salsa

MANUFACTURER/DISTRIBUTOR   VARIETY

Salt-free Seasoning Mixtures

These mixes are made with no added salt, but they do contain a small amount of natural sodium. They are made of dehydrated vegetables and spices. Watch for added salt and oils in any seasoning mixes you buy.

Alberto-Culver Co.	Mrs. Dash (Low Pepper-No Garlic, Extra Spicy, Original Blend, etc.)
Modern Products	Vegit-All Purpose Seasoning Onion Magic Natural Seasoning
Parsley Patch	All Purpose Mexican Blend
Maine Coast Sea Vegetables	Sea Seasonings (Dulse with Garlic, Nori with Ginger, etc.)
Estee Corp.	Seasoning Sense (Mexican, Italian)
Hain Pure Food Co.	Chili Seasoning Mix
Bernard Jensen Products	Broth or Seasoning Special Vegetable Mix

Baking Ingredients

These contain no aluminum and a minimum of additives.

The Rumford Co.	Rumford Baking Powder
Sandoz Nutrition	Featherweight Baking Powder
Ener-G Foods	Egg Replacer (a binder for baking)
Eden Foods	Kuzu Root Starch Agar Agar

Hot Drinks

These contain no caffeine or other strong herbs.

MANUFACTURER/DISTRIBUTOR   VARIETY

Hot Drinks (continued)

Many manufacturers	Noncaffeinated teas
Modern Products	Sipp
Libby, McNeill & Libby	Pero
Worthington Foods	Kaffree Roma
Richter Bros.	Cafix
General Foods Corp.	Postum
J. Intra-World Grain Prod.	Café du Grain

Canned and Bottled Beans and Vegetables

These products contain no added fats or oils and are low in sodium and preservatives. The cans are made of metals that leach into the foods unless they are coated. Glass jars, of course, have no metal.

Eden Foods	Great Northern Beans (glass jars) Pinto Beans (glass jars) Adzuki Beans (glass jars)
Whole Earth	Baked Beans
Health Valley Foods	Boston Baked Beans
Hain Pure Food Co.	Spicy Vegetarian Homestyle Chili
Bush Bros. & Co.	Bush's Deluxe Vegetarian Beans
Brazos Products	Cajun Bean Dip
S & W Fine Foods	Maple Syrup Beans Deli-Style Bean Salad Mixed Bean Salad (bottled) Dill Garden Salad Succotash Garden Style Pasta Salad (bottled)

MANUFACTURER/DISTRIBUTOR   VARIETY

Canned and Bottled Beans and Vegetables (continued)

Little Bear Organic Foods	Bearitos (Chili, Black Bean Dip)
American Home Food Products	Salad Bar (Marinated Medley, Three-Bean Salad, Garbanzo Beans, Kidney Beans)
Del Monte	Dennison's Chili Beans in Chili Gravy
Beatrice/Hunt-Wesson	Rosarita No Fat Refried Beans
Guiltless Gourmet	Bean Dips (bottled)
Walnut Acres	Garbanzo Beans Pinto Beans
Stop & Shop Supermarket Co.	Chick Peas
H.J. Heinz	Vegetarian Beans in Tomato Sauce
Trader Joe's	Spicy Black Bean Dip (bottled)

Canned Tomato Products

These products contain no added salt. If they are too bland, add salt at the table if your health permits. Metals leach from cans.

Health Valley Foods	Tomato Sauce (coated lead-free can)
Del Monte	Tomato Sauce (No Salt Added) Original Style Stewed Tomatoes with Onions, Celery, Green Peppers (No Salt Added) Tomato Paste
Beatrice/Hunt-Wesson	No Salt Added Tomato Paste No Salt Added Tomato Sauce No Salt Added Stewed Tomatoes No Salt Added Whole Tomatoes

Canned Tomatoe Products (continued)

Contadina Foods	Tomato Puree Tomato Paste
Pet	Progresso (Tomato Paste, Tomato Puree)
Eden Foods	Crushed Tomatoes (No Salt Added)
Trader Joe's	Tomato Sauce
S & W Fine Foods	No Salt Added Ready-Cut Peeled Tomatoes
Ital Trade, USA	Pomi (Strained Tomatoes, Chopped Tomatoes)
Walnut Acres	Tomato Puree Tomatoes

Canned Fruit Products

These contain just plain fruit and maybe some fruit juice, with no added sugars or syrups. Metals leach from cans.

Dole Packaged Foods Co.	Pineapple Chunks (in unsweetened juice) Crushed Pineapple (in unsweetened juice) Pineapple Slices (in unsweetened juice)
S & W Fine Foods	Nutradiet (Sliced Peaches, Grapefruit, Apricot Halves, Pear Halves, Sliced Peaches, Peach Halves) Mandarin Oranges (Natural Style, in its own juice) Grapefruit (Natural Style, in its own juice)

Canned Fruit Products (continued)

MANUFACTURER/DISTRIBUTOR	VARIETY
Tri Valley Growers	Libby's Lite (Sliced Peaches, Pear Halves)
Del Monte	Fruit Naturals (Diced Peaches, Mixed Fruit)

Acceptable Milk Substitutes

These are dairy free and low in natural vegetable fat. They should not to be used as beverages but on cereals and in cooking.

Grainaissance	Amazake Rice Drink
Eden Foods	Edensoy Vanilla Soy Milk
Sovex Natural foods	Better Than Milk? Light
Health Valley Foods	Soy Moo (low fat) Fat-Free Soy Moo
Vitasoy U.S.A.	Vitasoy Light—Original 1%
Westbrae Natural Foods	West Soy Lite (1% fat) Plain

Richer Foods

These richer foods are high in simple sugar and/or salt. Some caution must be used in adding these foods to your diet. Use sparingly!

Fruit Snacks

These are made of pure fruit, but are concentrated in calories and simple sugars. They have all been processed without sulphur dioxide (SO_2).

Sunfield	Nature's Choice Real Fruit Bars
Barbara's Bakery	Apples (and that's all)

MANUFACTURER/DISTRIBUTOR	VARIETY

Fruit Snacks (continued)

Stretch Island Fruit — Tropical Fruit Ripples (Mandarin Cherry, Banana)
Fruit Leather

Fruit Candies

Panda Factory — All Natural Bar

Sokensha Co. — Plum Candy

Erewhon — Plum Sweets
Cinnamon Sweets

Edward & Sons Trading Co. — Natural Temptations Rice Malt Candies

Cookies

Health Valley — Fat-Free Cookies (Raspberry, Raspberry Fruit Centers, Raisin Oatmeal, Apple Spice, and others)
Fat-Free Jumbo Fruit Bars (Apricot, Oat Bran Raisin Cinnamon, and others)

Natures Warehouse — Wheat-Free Cookies (Caramel Crisp, Raspberry)

Heaven Scent Natural Foods — Cookies (Mountain Berry, Old Fashioned Raisin)

Auburn Farms — Fat-Free Jammers

R.W. Frookies — Fat-Free All Natural Cookies

Trader Joe's — Very Berry Cookies

Lady J Inc. — Oatmeal Date Lites

MANUFACTURER/DISTRIBUTOR   VARIETY

Jellies, Jams, and Syrups

These have no added sugar, corn syrup, or other sugars, and few preservatives.

Clearbrook Farms	Fruit Spreads
M. Polaner	All Fruit (Jams)
Robertson Foods International	Pure Fruit Conserve
The J.M. Smucker Co.	Smucker's Simply Fruit (Red Raspberry, Strawberry, Blueberry, etc.)
Sorrell Ridge Farm	Sorrell Ridge Fruit Only (Apricot, Grape, etc.)
Knudsen & Sons	All Fruit Fancy Fruit Spreads (Concord Grape, Blueberry, Cranberry, etc.) Syrups (Raspberry, Boysenberry, Fruit N' Maple, Blueberry, Strawberry)
Shady Maple Farms	Maple Syrup
Many manufacturers	Honey
Westbrae Natural Foods	Brown Rice Syrup
Eden Foods	Barley Malt
Spring Tree Corp.	Pure Maple Syrup
Anderson's	Pure Maple Syrup
Camp	Pure Maple Syrup
Kozlowski Family	Apple Chutney Fruit Jams

MANUFACTURER/DISTRIBUTOR	VARIETY

Jellies, Jams, and Syrups (continued)

Lundberg Family Farms	Sweet Dreams Brown Rice Syrup
Timber Crest Farms	Dried Tomato Chutney
Nature's Harvest	Kiwi Preserve

Barbecue Sauces and Catsups

These sauces contain no added fats or oils, but most have salt and sugar, and some have preservatives.

Beatrice/Hunt-Wesson	Hunt's All Natural Thick & Rich Barbecue Sauce
Ridg's Finer Foods	Bull's Eye Original Barbecue Sauce Robbie's Sauce (Barbecue—mild and hot, Sweet & Sour Hawaiian Style) Ketchup
Hain Pure Food Co.	Catsup
Kingsford Products	K.C. Masterpiece Original Sauce
Mrs. Renfro's	Mrs. Renfro's Barbecue Sauce
Westbrae Natural Foods	Fruit Sweetened Catsup Unsweetened Un-Ketchup
Health Valley Foods	Catch-Up Tomato Table Sauce
Ventre Packing Co.	Enrico's Ketchup
Pure & Simple	Johnson's Ketchup
Beatrice/Hunt-Wesson	No Salt Added Tomato Ketchup
The Mayhaw Tree	Barbeque Sauce
Tim's Gourmet Foods	Tim's Barbecue Sauce

Ice Desserts

These are made from fruit and concentrated fruit juice, with no added dairy products (whey) or oils.

Dole Packaged Foods Co.	Fruit Sorbet (no dairy products) Fruit N' Juice Bars Dole Sun Tops—Real Fruit Juice Bars
Frozfruit Corp.	Frozfruit (Strawberry, Raspberry, Lemon, Canteloupe, Lime, Orange, Cherry, Pineapple)
The J.M. Smucker Co.	Fruitage Premium Frozen Dessert (Raspberry)

Rich, High-fat Packaged and Canned Products

Soy Milks

These are high-fat nondairy milks made from soybeans. You can make them healthier, and at the same time more palatable, by diluting one part soy milk with two to three parts water. Avoid those soy milks with added oils.

Ener-G Foods	Pure Soyquick
Health Valley Foods	Soy Moo
Eden Foods	Edensoy (other than vanilla)
Mitoku Co. Ltd.	Supersoy
Wholesome & Hearty	White Almond Beverage
Pacific Foods of Oregon	Organic Soy Beverage
Westbrae Natural Foods	Westsoy Plus

MANUFACTURER/DISTRIBUTOR	VARIETY

Soy Yogurt

Soyen Natural	Soya Latté (nondairy yogurt)
White Wave	Dairyless Yogurt

Tofu "Ice Cream"

Tofutti Brands	Lite Lite Tofutti (Vanilla)

Casein-free Soy Cheeses

Soyco Foods	Soymage (Cheddar Style, Mozzarella Style, Jalapeño Style)

Burger Mixes with Tofu

Fantastic Foods	Tofu Burger Mix
Sunfield Foods	Lite Chef Country Barbecue
Fantastic Foods	Tofu Scrambler Mix
Sahara Natural Foods	Gyros Greek Classics

Tofu, Nuts, Nut Butters, Seeds, Seed Spreads, Avocados, and Olives

These are all naturally very high in fat. Olives are usually high in salt also. Many nuts are cooked in oils and salted—don't buy these. Nut butters, such as peanut butter, should contain only the nuts, and maybe some salt. They should contain no preservatives, and should not have undergone processing, such as hydrogenization, which keeps the spread in a more solid consistency at room temperature. Some health-food stores will grind fresh nuts into nut butters for you. In this case there will be no added salt—only ground nuts. Seed spreads, such as tahini, should be made with pure sesame seeds. You can dilute nut and seed spreads with water. (Blend equal amounts of water and nut or seed butter in a food processor or blender.)

Help us update this list. Please send packages and package labels from products that make eating healthier and easier. This list was compiled in June 1992.

For an updated package list send with SASE to:

McDougalls
P.O. Box 14039
Santa Rosa, CA 95402

Challenge #5: Cooking Techniques

SOLUTIONS

Cook Without Oil

While leaving out the oil improves the taste of a food, you will have to find ways to replace the moisture and other qualities that oil provides. Almost all of the recipes you will start with have oil in one form or another as a prominent ingredient—unless they are from a McDougall book.

SAUTÉING

To sauté implies the use of butter or oil. But sautéing McDougall style eliminates these fats and instead uses liquids that give taste without damaging your health. Surprisingly, plain water makes an excellent sautéing liquid. It prevents foods from sticking to the pan and still allows vegetables to brown and cook. Browned onions, for example, take on an excellent flavor and color when sautéed in this fashion and can be used alone or mixed with other vegetables for a dish with a distinctive taste. Place 1½ cups of chopped onion in a large nonstick frying pan with 1 cup of water. Cook over medium heat, stirring occasionally, until the liquid evaporates and the onion begins to stick to the bottom of the pan. Continue to stir for a minute, then add another ½ cup of water, loosening the browned bits from the bottom of the pan. Cook until the liquid evaporates again. Repeat this procedure one or two more times, until the onion (or other vegetable) is as browned as you like. You can also use this technique to brown carrots, green peppers, garlic, potatoes, shallots, zucchini, and many other vegetables, alone or mixed.

For more flavor try sautéing in:

Soy sauce or tamari
Red or white wine (alcoholic or nonalcoholic)
Sherry (alcoholic or nonalcoholic)
Rice vinegar or balsalmic vinegar
Tomato juice
Lemon or lime juice
Salsa
Worcestershire sauce

For even more flavor, herbs and spices, such as ginger, dry mustard, horseradish and garlic, can be added.

BAKING

To eliminate oil in baking is a real challenge, because oil keeps baked goods moist and soft. Replace the oil called for in your recipe with half the amount of another moist food, such as applesauce, mashed bananas, mashed potatoes, mashed pumpkin, tomato sauce, soft (silken) tofu, or soy yogurt (but remember, tofu and soy yogurt are high-fat foods).

Cakes and muffins made without oil will be a little heavier. For a lighter texture, use carbonated water instead of tap water in baking recipes. Be sure to test cakes and muffins at the end of the baking time by inserting a toothpick or cake tester to see if it comes out clean. Sometimes oil-free cakes and muffins may need to be baked longer than the directions advise, depending on the weather or the altitude at which you live.

Rely on Packaged Support for McDougall Cooking

There are several packaged products that you will find very helpful in your cooking. They serve as substitutes for unhealthy ingredients, such as eggs, dairy products, gelatin, and oils.

Egg Replacer

Eliminating high-cholesterol, high-fat eggs from your diet means that you need a good binding agent for many recipes. A flour product called Ener-G Egg Replacer fills this role very effectively in baking. Most natural-foods stores carry this product. (Or you can order it directly from the company by writing to Ener-G Foods, Inc., PO Box 84487, Seattle, WA 98124, or calling 800-331-5222.)

To achieve the best results with this product, mix it with water according to the package directions, then beat until very frothy, using a whisk, electric beater, or blender. Ener-G will not make anything resembling scrambled eggs. It is for use in baked goods only.

Agar-Agar

Agar-agar is a natural vegetable "gelatin" product made from sea vegetables, sold as flakes, powder, or bars.* It is sold in most natural-food stores, either as flakes or in powder form. Manufacturers use it to thicken salad dressings, some ice creams, puddings, jellies, and candies. You can use it to gel liquids: Use 1½ tablespoons of flakes or ¾ teaspoon of powder to gel 1 cup of liquid. Use less to thicken a homemade dressing slightly.

Emes Kosher Gelatin

Emes is a natural vegetable "gelatin" used to thicken salad dressings and gel liquids. Use 1 tablespoon to gel 1¾ cups of liquid and slightly less for thickening dressings. Emes may be found in some natural-food stores or it may be ordered directly by writing to Emes Kosher Products, 4138-42 West Roosevelt Road, Chicago, IL 60624.

---

*Real gelatin is a mixture of proteins extracted by boiling the skin, bones, horns, and hoofs of animals.

GUAR GUM POWDER

Guar gum powder is a natural vegetable "gelatin" used as a salad-dressing thickener. One product, called Guar-Aid Powder, manufactured by Twin Lab, can be found in many natural-foods stores. Use between ½ and 1 teaspoon per cup of dressing. Allow the mixture to stand for an hour or longer. This product is useful also for thickening sauces to a spreading consistency. Guar gum can be purchased in most natural-food stores.

SOY MILK

Soy milk is made from soybeans and water with a sweetener sometimes added. Regular soy milk contains 5 grams of fat per serving (45 percent fat). Low-fat soy milks, labeled *lite* soy milks, contain only 2 grams of fat per serving (18 percent fat). To reduce the amount of fat even more, and at the same time thin out the strong taste of soy, you can dilute soy milk with an equal amount of water. Soy milk replaces cow's milk on a cup-per-cup exchange in all recipes. Soy milk is not recommended as a beverage because of its high fat content.

RICE MILK

Rice milk has a lighter, sweeter taste than soy milk and is much lower in fat. Made from cooked fresh fermented brown rice, it is white in color and has a consistency resembling cow's milk. Rice milk can be found in most natural-food stores or can be made at home. (See page 90.)

Choose Cookware Carefully

An easy way to eliminate oil from your cooking is to use nonstick pans. Acceptable materials for cookware include glass, stainless steel, iron, nonstick pans and bakeware (such as Dupont's Silverstone or Teflon), silicone-coated bakeware (such as Baker's Secret), and porcelain. A light oiling when you first get a Teflon or Silverstone implement will help to prevent sticking. Cast-iron pans and woks should be oiled before they're first used and then "seasoned" by heating. (Follow the manufacturer's instructions.)

When buying cookware you need to pay most attention to the surface that your foods will be in contact with, because your food will inevitably pick up molecules from the utensils' surface. Aluminum cookware should be avoided because of the association between aluminum ingestion and Alzheimer's disease. (If you're stuck with an aluminum pan or pot, punch holes in the bottom and plant flowers in it.) For cake pans, loaf pans, and baking sheets, you can place parchment paper between the metal and your food. Parchment paper, which can be found in most grocery stores, also keeps food from sticking to the surface of pans. It can also be used under (or over) aluminum foil, in order to keep the aluminum from coming in contact with the food. Place a layer of parchment paper over the food in a baking dish, then cover with foil, turning the edges over the pan to hold in the steam.

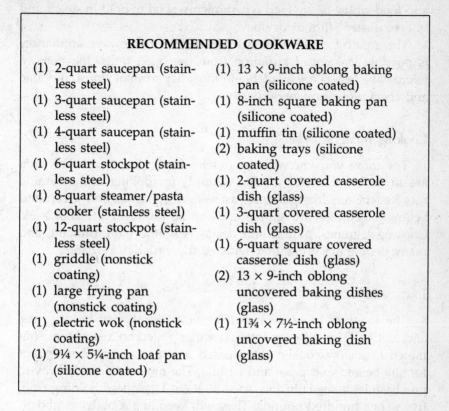

RECOMMENDED COOKWARE

(1) 2-quart saucepan (stainless steel)

(1) 3-quart saucepan (stainless steel)

(1) 4-quart saucepan (stainless steel)

(1) 6-quart stockpot (stainless steel)

(1) 8-quart steamer/pasta cooker (stainless steel)

(1) 12-quart stockpot (stainless steel)

(1) griddle (nonstick coating)

(1) large frying pan (nonstick coating)

(1) electric wok (nonstick coating)

(1) 9¼ × 5¼-inch loaf pan (silicone coated)

(1) 13 × 9-inch oblong baking pan (silicone coated)

(1) 8-inch square baking pan (silicone coated)

(1) muffin tin (silicone coated)

(2) baking trays (silicone coated)

(1) 2-quart covered casserole dish (glass)

(1) 3-quart covered casserole dish (glass)

(1) 6-quart square covered casserole dish (glass)

(2) 13 × 9-inch oblong uncovered baking dishes (glass)

(1) 11¾ × 7½-inch oblong uncovered baking dish (glass)

If vegetables stick while cooking in a pan or baking tray, let them cool for 5 to 10 minutes and they will loosen easily. Cooling will also loosen muffins from tins.

Use a Microwave Oven

Ever since the introduction of the microwave oven, some people have been suspicious of "nuked" foods. However, tests on the foods show excellent nutrient content and no significant increase in harmful byproducts from microwave heating when compared to conventional oven cooking. We use a microwave mostly for boiling small quantities of water, reheating leftovers, thawing vegetables, and cooking potatoes, but sauces, stews, casseroles, and vegetables also cook well in a microwave oven. Microwave cooking is fast and convenient. Less liquid is needed and cooking times are reduced, compared to oven cooking. But you must stir or rotate foods often, and foods must be covered when microwaved to hold in steam and to cook faster without drying.

The greatest concern about the safety of microwave appliances is possible leakage of radiation from damaged units. Inexpensive microwave testers are available in most department stores. Buy one and check your unit periodically.

Cooking Basic Starches

The more you know about starchy foods, the more likely you are to cook successful meals. Methods for boiling and steaming root vegetables, like potatoes, as well as squashes and green and yellow vegetables, are simple and can be found in any cookbook. Cooking legumes, grains, and pastas is a little more difficult, and many people are unfamiliar with all the varieties available.

LEGUMES

The legumes category includes many varieties of beans, peas, and lentils. They are easy to cook, either boiled on a stovetop, simmered in a slow cooker, or prepared in a pressure cooker (except for soy beans, split peas, and lentils). The most economical way to purchase legumes is in the dried state, in large bags holding from five to one hundred pounds. They will keep in a cool dry cupboard for months. Before cooking, sort legumes by hand, removing stones and any discolored seeds.

BOILING LEGUMES

Place the legumes in water (see the following chart for amounts) in a large pot and bring to a boil. Reduce the heat, cover, and cook at a gentle boil for the recommended time (see the accompanying table). The longer you cook them, the softer legumes become, the more indigestible carbohydrates are broken down, and the less trouble you will have with bowel gas. Salads call for firmer beans, cooked just to the point of being tender. Legumes for soups and spreads need to be cooked longer. Never add salt while cooking—it makes beans tough.

Cooking Times for Legumes

BEANS (1 CUP)	WATER (CUPS)	TIME (HOURS)	YIELD (CUPS)
Adzuki beans	4	1½	2
Black beans	4	1½	2
Black-eyed peas	3	1	2
Garbanzo beans	4	3	2
Kidney beans	3	2	2
Lentils*	3	1	2
Split peas*	3	1	2
Lima beans	3	1½	2
Pinto beans	3	2½	2
White beans	3	2	2

*Do not need presoaking.

Cooking times can be reduced by two methods:

1. Soak the beans overnight in enough water to cover them and 2 to 3 extra inches. After soaking, drain off the water and cook according to the instructions above, but reduce the cooking time by 1 hour.

2. To save both time and energy, bring the beans to a boil with the amount of water suggested in the table for 2 minutes. Remove from the heat, cover, and let rest for 1 hour. Do not drain. Then proceed with the directions above, but reduce the cooking time by ½ hour.

If you use the longer cooking times with these methods, you will end up with more thoroughly cooked beans.

SLOW-COOKING LEGUMES

Slow cookers are convenient, and they conserve electricity. Place the legumes in the slow cooker, and cover with the appropriate amount of water (see the accompanying table). Cook for 6 to 8 hours on high or 10 to 12 hours on low.

PRECOOKED LEGUMES

Beans and lentils can be bought already cooked and packaged in bottles or cans. Black-eyed peas can be found cooked and frozen. In time, more of these convenient packaged foods will be found in the markets. While the precooked packaged varieties are more expensive, they are also more convenient. The extra cost must be balanced against your savings in energy bills and against the value of your time.

Look for beans bottled or canned in water only or in water and salt. Drain and rinse the beans before using them in a recipe. Use them just as you would dried beans you cooked at home. Some recipes require dried beans, however, because the cooking liquid is the basis of a sauce. Canned and bottled beans may always be used in recipes calling for cooked beans.

The Unmentionable Gas

By about the fourth day of each McDougall Program at St. Helena Hospital and Health Center, the participants have become close friends. As they loosen up with one another, they begin to discuss a noticeable side effect of the diet. They make jokes like, "When we walk, we talk," or "Have you heard a good McBugle lately?" I must admit that one unavoidable problem with the diet I recommend is the production of more gas.

Abundant intestinal gas, called flatulence, when released from the lower bowel can be a social problem. On the average this gas, called *flatus*, is passed ten to twenty times a day, and the volume can vary from twelve to eighty ounces of gas a day on the usual American diet. You can assume the upper levels in frequency and volume for anyone on the McDougall Program. Accumulation of this gas in the gut can be accompanied by abdominal cramps— usually relieved by passing the gas.

The gas is produced by the action of intestinal bacteria on foods. Carbohydrates that have not been absorbed in the process of normal digestion by enzymes in the small intestine are moved undigested into the large intestine (colon), where bacteria break them down by the process known as *fermentation*. Five gases—nitrogen, oxygen, hydrogen, carbon dioxide, and small amounts of methane—account for 99 percent of bowel gas. These gases are odorless. The strong odor of bowel gas comes primarily from products of bacterial putrefaction of animal proteins and fats in the large intestine. Avoiding animal products in your diet will mean cleaner and fresher air in your immediate vicinity.

The most common source of undigested carbohydrate is lactose from dairy products, such as milk and yogurt (cheeses contain little lactose). The second biggest gas-producing foods are legumes, be they the beans that accompany a hot dog, or those in a low-fat vegetarian chili. They contain two relatively indigestible sugars, raffinose and stachyose, that end up in the large intestine, where they are decomposed into gases by bowel bacteria.

I submit two comments in defense of my Program: First, when human beings were designed a few million years ago, no confining walls hemmed them in. Second, bowel gases produced from a starch-based diet are much less malodorous than are those from a diet rich in proteins. For people following the McDougall Program, the adjustment to high-fiber foods occurs in time, and the amount of gas produced diminishes in about two weeks. Much of this adjustment comes as a consequence of changes in the kinds and numbers of bowel bacteria.

SOLUTIONS TO THE EMBARRASSMENT OF GAS

Avoid Gassy Foods: Milk products are troublesome for most non-Caucasian people (Asians, Blacks, Hispanics, Indians, Eskimos, etc.), who can't digest lactose; about 20 percent of Caucasians also have this trouble. All legumes—beans, peas, lentils, etc.—bother people of all races indiscriminately. Some individuals have trouble with onions, bagels, pretzels, prunes, apricots, cabbage, carrots, celery, green peppers, broccoli, cauliflower, bananas, Brussels sprouts, and wheat germ. But the list of offenders depends on personalized sensitivities and could include almost any food.

Cook Foods Thoroughly: Almost everyone seems to have a method of "de-gassing" beans. Many cooks claim to have inherited the secret process from an authoritative grandmother. Thus, I've heard some say, "Add potatoes to beans during cooking," while others insist, "Discard the rinse water." I haven't found any of these methods to be of benefit. Soaking helps, whether or not you discard the original rinse water, simply because soaking starts the breakdown of the carbohydrates and assists cooking. Thorough cooking helps by breaking down indigestible complex carbohydrates into simpler, more digestible forms.

Sprout Legumes: One reliable way to "de-gas" legumes is to sprout them first: Cover them with water for twelve hours. Drain off the water, and lay moist paper towels on the bottom of a baking dish. Spread the legumes on the moist towels, and let them sprout for the next twelve hours. When you notice tiny white shoots (1/16 inch) beginning to appear, they are ready to cook. The tiny plant is utilizing the indigestible sugars for growth. Needless to say, beans will take less time to cook after sprouting.

Use Beano: A new product on the market, Beano, contains enzymes that are capable of breaking down the indigestible sugars in beans, peas, and lentils. You add a couple of drops to the first bite of food, and then you can eat the rest without the problem of bowel gas. (Or so the label says. . . .)

Use Activated Charcoal: For those who have found no other solution and need help, activated charcoal, sold in 260-mg capsules, has been shown to relieve discomfort and reduce the volume of gas. Activated charcoal for this purpose is popular in India and Europe and has only recently been gaining acceptance in the United States. The exact mechanism of action is unknown, but the charcoal may inhibit gas-producing bacteria, enhance bacterial consumption of gas, or act by absorbing hydrogen and carbon dioxide. (Note: Charcoal absorbs and inactivates many substances, including medications.)

GRAINS

Rice is the most familiar grain to Americans and the most commonly consumed food in the world. A large variety of other whole grains are available to choose from. Experimenting with them will pay off, because you will discover new favorite foods that rate high on both the taste and the nutrition scale.

Cooking Times for Grains

WHOLE GRAINS (1 CUP)	WATER (CUPS)	TIME (MIN.)	YIELD (CUPS)
barley	2	60	3
buckwheat	2	15	2½
bulgur wheat	2	15	2½
cornmeal	4	30	4
millet	3	45	3½
quinoa	2	15	3
rice (brown)	2	60	3
rye	2	60	2½
wheat berries	3	120	3

Boiling is the usual way to cook these grains. Bring the appropriate quantity of water (see the accompanying table) to a boil in a saucepan. Slowly add the grain. Return the water to a boil, cover, reduce the heat to low, and cook for the amount of time specified, or until the water has been absorbed. Do not stir. For fluffier texture, allow the grain to rest, uncovered, for 15 minutes after cooking. This helps dry the grain. For a variation, try a mix of two or more grains, or use a vegetable stock instead of water. Grains can be cooked more easily and more reliably in a rice cooker. Unfortunately, most brands of rice cookers have aluminum insert bowls. To reduce the contact of your grain with this possibly neurotoxic metal, you can use a stainless-steel bowl inserted in the aluminum bowl. Better yet, National (made by Panasonic) and Hitachi make rice cookers with a nonstick coating and stainless-steel covers, protecting your food from exposure to aluminum.

Bulgur may also be prepared by pouring boiling water over it in a bowl. Cover the bowl with a kitchen towel and wait for 1 hour. Pour the bulgur and water into a mesh strainer and press out excess water.

PASTAS

Pastas are made from flour and water. Wheat flour is most commonly used, but there are combinations with other grain flours. Some pastas are entirely wheat free, like those made from quinoa, corn, and rice. Manufactured flours have had some of the fiber removed in the processing, and some of the more refined varieties should be considered "white" flours. The 100 percent durum semolina pastas have the most familiar flavor and body of the "white"-flour pastas. The flour with the highest content of dietary fiber is whole-wheat flour, and you will notice this by the coarser texture of whole-wheat pasta. The most important criterion when choosing a pasta is to find one made of only flour and water, containing no egg or oil. Good-quality pasta makes a very palatable companion to simple, oil-free sauces.

KINDS OF PASTA

Artichoke pasta—made from dehydrated artichoke and whole-wheat flours

Buckwheat soba—made from buckwheat and whole-wheat flours

Corn pasta—made from cornmeal

Quinoa pasta—made from corn, quinoa, and sesame flours

Rice pasta—made from ground brown rice

Soy pasta—made from soy and wheat flours

Spinach pasta—made from ground dehydrated spinach and re-fined whole-wheat flour

Tomato pasta—made from ground dehydrated tomatoes and re-fined whole-wheat flour

Whole-wheat pasta—made from whole-wheat flour

COOKING PASTA

For 1 pound of pasta, you need about 4 to 5 quarts of water. Do not add oil or salt to the water. One pound of pasta will serve four people with normal appetites. Bring the water to a rolling boil. Drop the pasta into the water; it is not necessary to break long strands; they will soften and sink into the water. Cook at a rolling boil, uncovered, stirring occasionally. Test for doneness after 5 minutes by biting into a piece. Pasta should be firm, never soggy. Cooking time will vary but should be no longer than 12 minutes. When the pasta is done, drain it in a colander, rinse it with cool water to help prevent sticking, and put it in a bowl. Serve immediately, or mix with sauce before serving. (Mixing with a sauce keeps strands of pasta from sticking together as they cool.)

Challenge #6: Seasoning Foods

SOLUTIONS

Spice Your Foods According to Personal Preference

You should use the recipes in this book and those in the other McDougall books as guidelines only. You may prefer to add more or less spice. We learned about individual tastes through years of counseling people. One person would tell Mary, "Your food is so bland. Every time I make a dish I have to double the spice." The very next person would ask Mary why she uses so much spice.

Mary has tried to flavor her recipes to satisfy the average palate. (However, this moderate seasoning approach is subject to Mary's interpretation. For example, she happens to love curry and I do not. Fortunately, over the years, my tastes have changed enough to where I can enjoy many of her Indian and Thai dishes.)

When deciding whether to use fresh herbs or dried ones, consider how long the food is going to cook. For a long cooking time, dried herbs are generally best. For a short cooking time, use fresh herbs, if they're available, to really appreciate the flavors these can add to foods. For equal flavor you will need more fresh herbs than dried ones, because the dried ones are more concentrated. In time, however, dried herbs lose their potency.

Certain combinations of herbs, spices, and other seasonings are identified with ethnic dishes. You can take advantage of these to vary recipes and create new ones.

Mexican	*Italian*	*Asian*
Salsa	Parsley	Soy sauce
Chili powder	Basil	Ginger
Cumin	Oregano	Dry mustard
Cilantro	Garlic	Garlic

Greek	*Indian*
Lemon juice	Turmeric
Cinnamon	Pepper
Cumin	Cilantro
Pepper	Cumin

Place the Salt Shaker on the Table

Salt is the taste missed most when people switch to a healthful diet. If you feel your food is bland, then salt is what you are missing. Even if you never salted your food in the past, the amount in the prepared and packaged foods you used to eat was substantially more than is available in an unsalted starch-based diet, which generally provides only 100 to 300 mg daily. The way to improve the taste of your food is to add salt, so the salt-appreciating taste buds on the tip of your tongue will be delightfully stimulated. Delightfully, please note, not dangerously!

The best way to keep salt intake under control is to avoid cooking with salt as much as possible. Salt sprinkled on the surface of a food comes in direct contact with the tongue, providing the greatest pleasure for the smallest amount used. A few light sprinkles of salt will be enough for most people. Each half teaspoon of salt adds only 1,150 mg of sodium. This generous amount used daily will please most people's palates. Altogether this amounts to 1,450 mg a day at most—550 mg less than the 2,000 mg "low-sodium" diet served to patients dying of "heart disease" in your local hospital's intensive care unit. To bring the sodium intake up to the daily American average of more than 5,000 mg, you would have to pour more than 2 teaspoons of salt on the surface of your starch-based meals every day. This amount of salt would make the food unpalatable for most people.

If at first your food still tastes a little bland, be patient. You will soon adjust to less salt and new flavors. Appreciation of the salty taste of foods is a learned behavior. Enjoying a lower salt intake is simply a matter of changing your habitual use and exposing your taste buds to lesser amounts. Satisfaction generally begins in about four days.

NOTES ON SALT IN RECIPES

Salt is allowed in a few of our recipes as an option, when it really improves taste. Most of the recipes are deliciously spiced and will not need to have any salt added in cooking or at the table, especially after you adjust your tongue and palate.

These recipes do not call for low-sodium tomato products because most people can tolerate the amount of salt used in canning. If you are salt sensitive, however, you will need to purchase the low-sodium varieties. For salt-free alternatives, use chopped fresh tomatoes in place of canned tomatoes, and in place of tomato sauce, puree fresh tomatoes in a blender.

Use Soy Sauce

Soy sauce provides a flavorful alternative to plain table salt. Don't be fooled into thinking there is no sodium in soy sauce, however. The regular variety has 800 mg of sodium per tablespoon, the low-salt varieties 500 mg per tablespoon. When choosing a brand of soy sauce, avoid the ingredient monosodium glutamate (MSG). Many people have reactions to this substance, and, of course, it represents another source of sodium. Soy sauce is also sold under the name tamari, which is more strongly flavored. The taste of soy sauce will vary, depending upon the producer. You will probably develop a preference for one brand.

Sweeteners May Save the Dish

Sweet is the other pleasurable taste appreciated by the sensory buds on the tip of the tongue. You may wish to take advantage of this by adding a small amount of sweetener to the surface of your oatmeal or other cereal. A teaspoon of cane sugar supplies only 16 calories. This small amount is unlikely to make a difference between gaining or losing weight. But those few sweet-tasting calories may be the difference that allows you to eat your cereal with pleasure. Other concentrated sweeteners include maple syrup, honey, molasses, brown sugar, and concentrated fruit juice.*

If you like (and can tolerate them without adverse effects) you may use artificial sweeteners, but I see little advantage to them, since sugar used in reasonable amounts does not cause obesity or poor health. If you use artificial sweeteners, apply them to the surface of your food for maximum taste.

Have Favorite Condiments on the Table

Having the right condiment or prepared sauce on the table can save the meal for family members not yet ecstatic about new dishes. Take advantage, as well, of the enjoyment provided by traditional sauces. (Make your own or use the many sauces in the packaged-and-canned products list on pages 42–69.)

---

*As far as nutrition is concerned, sugar is sugar. There is little difference between the nutritional content of honey, maple syrup, molasses, brown sugar, or white sugar. They are all simple carbohydrates, best described as "empty calories." They contain no fiber, protein, or fat and contribute little or nothing to vitamin and mineral needs. Artificial sweeteners have their drawbacks, too. They don't taste as good as natural sugars. They can cause unpleasant reactions, such as headaches, in some sensitive people. A few people claim even more severe reactions. When you understand that sugar is a minor health hazard, unless used in very large amounts, then you'll realize there is little reason to resort to artificial sweeteners.

CHAPTER 3

BREAKFASTS, BREADS, MUFFINS, AND SPREADS

The breakfast meal should be the easiest transition for you and your family (except for the milk). You already enjoy hot and cold cereals, breads, muffins, waffles, and pancakes. Most people can use small amounts of sweetener on these items, such as brown sugar on oatmeal, maple syrup on waffles and pancakes, and natural unsweetened jams on toast or muffins. The butter, cream, and milk have to be omitted for health reasons. Even so, most people will not feel the slightest bit deprived, because most of the pleasing taste from these items comes from the sweeteners' stimulation of the taste buds on the tip of the tongue (compare plain toast, pancakes, and waffles).

In place of milk, we have provided several delicious white liquids made from vegetable products. The banana and rice milks are very low in fat and should be the choice for those looking to lose weight and to avoid the strains on health caused by fat. The creamy-tasting cashew milk might be the best choice for children who can use a little extra fat for their energetic bodies.

Most bread recipes suggest unhealthy ingredients such as oil and milk. The recipes in this chapter show you it is possible to have great taste and good health (and the breads don't turn out like bricks). Bread machines have become very popular because they make a convenient, fresh-tasting product. Most of the recipes that come with the machines are a step or two away from being "McDougall legal." Oil-Free Stone-Ground Whole-Wheat Bread is a healthy bread designed to be made in a bread machine.

Breakfasts can be simple, like a bowl of cold cereal with store-bought rice milk, or a piece of toast with jam. However, some of you who are not so rushed in the morning will want to make an extra effort. Try French Toast, Wonderful "Buttermilk" Pancakes, and Hash-Brown Medley. There are also some nontraditional items like Breakfast Tortillas, or the East-West Breakfast made with rice and potatoes. What better time of the day to be adventuresome than the morning?

Breakfasts

Sunny Breakfast Couscous Cereal

SERVINGS: 4

PREPARATION TIME: 10 MINUTES

COOKING TIME: 5 TO 6 MINUTES IN MICROWAVE OVEN

¾ cup water
¼ cup fresh-squeezed orange juice
½ cup couscous
1 teaspoon finely grated orange zest
2 tablespoons finely chopped blanched almonds (optional)

1 tablespoon honey
1 tablespoon frozen apple juice concentrate
Dash ground cinnamon

Combine all of the ingredients in a 1-quart microwaveable casserole dish. Cover. Microwave on high until the liquid is absorbed and the couscous is tender, 5 to 6 minutes. Let stand, covered, for 1 minute more.

Multigrain Hot Cereal

SERVINGS: 2
PREPARATION TIME: 30 MINUTES
COOKING TIME: 30 MINUTES
RESTING TIME: 15 MINUTES

¼ cup long-grain brown rice
2 tablespoons barley
2 tablespoons millet
2 tablespoons rye

2 tablespoons wheat berries
6 dried apricots, chopped
2 cups water

Rinse the grains and soak them in water to cover for 30 minutes. Drain. Place the soaked grains in a rice cooker or a saucepan along with the apricots and 2 cups of water. Cook over low heat until the water is absorbed, about 17 minutes in a saucepan; a rice cooker will shut off automatically. Let rest for 15 minutes before serving.

Overnight Porridge

SERVINGS: 4
PREPARATION TIME: 5 MINUTES, PLUS OVERNIGHT REFRIGERATION
COOKING TIME: 6 TO 8 MINUTES; MICROWAVE TIME: 5 TO 7 MINUTES

½ cup bulghur
3 tablespoons rolled oats
1 tablespoon molasses or
brown rice syrup

⅓ cup mixed dried fruit
pieces or raisins
1½ cups water

Place all of the ingredients in a medium-sized bowl. Stir well. Cover and refrigerate overnight. Transfer to a saucepan or microwaveable dish.

Stove method: Cook over medium heat for 6 to 8 minutes, stirring frequently.

Microwave method: Cover with clear plastic wrap, vented at one corner. Microwave at 100 percent power for 5 to 7 minutes, stirring twice while heating.

Breakfast Rice

SERVINGS: 6
PREPARATION TIME: 5 MINUTES
COOKING TIME: 40 MINUTES
RESTING TIME: 10 MINUTES

1 cup long-grain brown rice   1 cup water
1 cup unsweetened apple   ½ cup raisins
   juice   ½ teaspoon ground cinnamon

Combine all of the ingredients in a saucepan. Bring to a boil, cover, reduce the heat, and cook for 40 minutes. Let rest for 10 minutes before serving.

This may also be made in a slow cooker overnight. Combine all of the ingredients and cook on low for 8 to 10 hours.

Rice Milk

SERVINGS: MAKES 1 QUART
PREPARATION TIME: 5 MINUTES (NEED COOKED RICE)

4 cups water   1 teaspoon vanilla extract
1 cup cooked long-grain   (optional)
   brown rice

Place all of the ingredients in a blender or food processor and process until smooth. Refrigerate. Shake before using.

For a smoother milk, pour through a strainer to remove some of the rice fibers.

Cashew Milk

SERVINGS: MAKES 1 QUART
PREPARATION TIME: 5 MINUTES

4 cups water   **¾ cup raw cashews, rinsed**

Place the water and cashews in a blender or food processor and process until smooth. Pour through a strainer. Refrigerate. Shake before using.

Banana Milk

SERVINGS: MAKES 1½ CUPS
PREPARATION TIME: 5 MINUTES

This milk is especially good over cereal.

1 banana, peeled and sliced   **½ teaspoon vanilla extract**
1 cup water   **(optional)**

Place all of the ingredients in a blender and process until smooth.

Fruity Golden Waffles

SERVINGS: 12
PREPARATION TIME: 15 MINUTES
COOKING TIME: 8 TO 10 MINUTES PER BATCH

4 cups rolled oats
⅓ cup whole-wheat flour
¼ cup chopped dates or
    raisins, or 2 tablespoons
    honey

½ teaspoon salt
5 cups water

Mix the oats, flour, dates, raisins or honey, and salt in a large bowl. Add the water to make a batter. Pour the batter into a blender in batches and blend until the consistency is smooth. (Or process all at once in a food processor.) Cook for 8 to 10 minutes in a waffle iron set on high.

Notes: 1. These freeze well.
2. You may omit the sweetener and use these as a base for beans or other savory sauces.

Waffles

SERVINGS: MAKES SEVEN 7-INCH WAFFLES
PREPARATION TIME: 10 MINUTES
RISING TIME: 30 TO 45 MINUTES
COOKING TIME: 5 TO 7 MINUTES PER BATCH

These are crisp and delicious. Serve them with Chunky Apple Syrup (page 95) or your favorite topping.

2½ cups warm water
2 cups whole-wheat pastry flour
2 tablespoons oat bran
2 tablespoons molasses or honey

1 tablespoon active dry yeast
½ teaspoon salt

Combine all of the ingredients in a large bowl. Stir with a spoon not more than fifty times, or until smooth. The batter will be thin but will thicken as it stands. Cover the bowl with a towel and place it in a warm place for 30 to 45 minutes, or until the batter is bubbly and thick. Bake in a nonstick waffle iron on low heat, 5 to 7 minutes. (The iron can be seasoned lightly with liquid lethicin or oil, if necessary.)

Variation: Fold two peeled and grated apples or two mashed bananas into the batter after it has risen and just before the waffles are baked.

Wonderful "Buttermilk" Pancakes

SERVINGS: MAKES TEN 4-INCH PANCAKES
PREPARATION TIME: 15 MINUTES
COOKING TIME: 1½ TO 2 MINUTES PER BATCH

One 6-ounce carton plain soy yogurt
⅓ cup water
1 teaspoon Ener-G Egg Replacer, well beaten with 2 tablespoons water

1 cup whole-wheat pastry flour
1 teaspoon baking powder
½ teaspoon baking soda
¼ teaspoon salt

Blend the yogurt, water, and Egg Replacer mixture thoroughly. Combine the remaining ingredients in a separate bowl. Add the dry ingredients to the wet ingredients and mix until moistened.

Cook on a nonstick griddle over medium heat until golden brown on both sides, about 2 minutes total.

French Toast

SERVINGS: 8
PREPARATION TIME: 5 MINUTES   COOKING TIME: 10 MINUTES PER BATCH

Serve these with maple syrup, applesauce, Chunky Apple Syrup (opposite page), or fruit.

½ pound soft tofu
1¼ cups water
1 teaspoon honey
¼ teaspoon vanilla extract

Pinch ground turmeric (for color)
8 slices whole-wheat or sourdough bread

Place the tofu, water, honey, vanilla, and turmeric in a blender or food processor and process until smooth. Transfer to a large bowl. Dip slices of bread into the mixture to coat both sides well. Cook on a dry nonstick griddle until brown on both sides.

Chunky Apple Syrup

SERVINGS: MAKES 2 CUPS
PREPARATION TIME: 10 MINUTES
COOKING TIME: 10 MINUTES

Serve this delicious topping over pancakes, waffles, hot cereal, or French toast.

1½ cups unsweetened apple
   juice
2½ teaspoons cornstarch
½ teaspoon brown sugar

⅛ teaspoon ground coriander
1 tart apple, peeled and
   diced

Combine the juice, cornstarch, sugar, and coriander in a saucepan. Cook, stirring, until the mixture thickens and turns clear. Remove from the heat.

Steam the diced apple over a small amount of water until softened, about 5 minutes. Add to the syrup. Serve warm.

Blueberry Sauce

SERVINGS: MAKES 2 CUPS
PREPARATION TIME: 5 MINUTES
COOKING TIME: 5 MINUTES

Serve this over pancakes, waffles, French toast, or hot cereal.

1 cup unsweetened
   pineapple juice
4 teaspoons cornstarch

1 cup blueberries, thawed
   frozen or fresh

Place the juice in a saucepan with the cornstarch. Cook, stirring, until thickened. Add the blueberries. Heat through. Serve warm.

Peach Sauce

SERVINGS: MAKES 3½ CUPS
PREPARATION TIME: 10 TO 20 MINUTES
COOKING TIME: 6 TO 8 MINUTES

Serve this over pancakes, waffles, French toast, or hot cereal.

3 peaches, peeled, or 3 cups
frozen peach slices,
thawed
1 cup fresh-squeezed orange
juice

2 tablespoons cornstarch
¼ teaspoon ground nutmeg

If using fresh peaches, slice two of them. Set aside. Coarsely chop
the remaining peach. For frozen fruit, set aside 2 cups.

Pour the orange juice into a blender. Add the chopped peach *or*
1 cup of the sliced frozen peaches. Blend until smooth. Pour into a
saucepan; add the cornstarch and nutmeg. Cook, stirring constantly, until thickened. Add the remaining sliced peaches. Heat
through. Serve warm.

Strawberry Sauce

SERVINGS: MAKES 2 CUPS
PREPARATION TIME: 5 MINUTES
COOKING TIME: 6 TO 8 MINUTES

Serve this over pancakes, waffles, French toast, or hot cereal.

1 cup unsweetened apple
juice
1 cup sliced strawberries,
thawed frozen or fresh

1 tablespoon cornstarch

Pour the juice into a blender and add ½ cup of the strawberries. Process until smooth. Pour into a saucepan. Add the cornstarch and stir until well mixed. Cook, stirring, until thickened. Add the remaining strawberries. Heat through and serve warm.

Pineapple-Banana Sauce

SERVINGS: MAKES 2 CUPS
PREPARATION TIME: 10 MINUTES
COOKING TIME: 5 TO 7 MINUTES

Serve this over pancakes, waffles, French toast, or hot cereal.

1½ cups unsweetened
    pineapple juice
2 tablespoons cornstarch
1 teaspoon fresh lemon
    juice

½ cup crushed pineapple in
    its own juice, drained
1 banana, peeled and sliced

Place the pineapple juice, cornstarch, and lemon juice in a saucepan. Cook, stirring, over medium heat until thickened. Remove from the heat and cool until lukewarm. Add the pineapple and banana and serve at once.

East-West Breakfast

SERVINGS: 4

PREPARATION TIME: 15 MINUTES (NEED COOKED RICE AND POTATOES)

COOKING TIME: 10 TO 12 MINUTES

1 medium onion, chopped	2 large boiled potatoes, peeled or unpeeled, and chopped
1 stalk celery, chopped	
⅓ cup chopped green bell pepper	1 cup cooked brown rice
	1 teaspoon ground cumin
½ cup water	1 tablespoon soy sauce

Sauté the onion, celery, and green pepper in ¼ cup of the water in a large nonstick frying pan for 5 minutes. Add the potatoes and the remaining ¼ cup water. Cook, stirring gently, until the vegetables are tender, about 5 minutes. Stir in the rice, cumin, and soy sauce. Cook, stirring, until the bottom browns lightly, about 2 minutes.

Hash-Brown Medley

SERVINGS: 4 TO 6

PREPARATION TIME: 20 MINUTES

COOKING TIME: 20 MINUTES

4 potatoes, peeled or unpeeled, cut into ¾-inch cubes	4 cloves garlic, sliced
	1 cup water
	2 cups thawed frozen or fresh corn
1 green bell pepper, chopped into large pieces	
1 onion, cut into cubes (separate the pieces)	1 large tomato, diced

Place the potatoes, green pepper, onion, and garlic in a nonstick frying pan with ½ cup of the water. Cook, stirring, over medium heat for 5 minutes. Add the remaining ½ cup water. Cover and continue to cook for another 10 minutes, stirring occasionally. Add the corn and tomato. Cook, stirring, for an additional 5 minutes.

Note: You can substitute frozen hash-brown potatoes for fresh potatoes in this recipe.

Country Potato Patties

SERVINGS: 4

PREPARATION TIME: 15 MINUTES (NEED COOKED POTATOES)
COOKING TIME: 10 MINUTES

3 large potatoes, peeled or unpeeled, boiled until soft

2 tablespoons finely chopped onion

2 tablespoons finely chopped celery

2 tablespoons finely chopped green bell pepper

2 tablespoons whole-wheat flour

1 tablespoon minced fresh parsley

Shred the potatoes in a food processor or with a grater. Combine with the remaining ingredients and shape into four patties. Cook on a nonstick griddle until browned on both sides, about 10 minutes.

Better Than Firesign Potatoes

SERVINGS: 2 TO 4
PREPARATION TIME: 10 MINUTES (NEED COOKED POTATOES)
COOKING TIME: 15 MINUTES

These were inspired by some breakfast potatoes we had at a restaurant on Lake Tahoe, called Firesign Cafe. We like this version better.

1 pound red potatoes (skins on), boiled until soft
1 small sweet onion, chopped
1 bunch scallions, finely chopped
Freshly ground pepper

Coarsely chop the cooked potatoes. Combine the potato, onion, and scallions. Place a small amount of water in a nonstick skillet. Add the vegetables; grind some fresh pepper over them. Cook, turning frequently with a spatula, until the potatoes brown slightly, about 15 minutes.

Breakfast Polenta with Orange-Maple Syrup

SERVINGS: 24
PREPARATION TIME: 5 MINUTES, PLUS OVERNIGHT CHILLING
COOKING TIME: 10 TO 12 MINUTES TO COOK POLENTA; 10 TO 12 MINUTES TO BROWN

2¾ cups fresh-squeezed orange juice
2½ cups water
1¼ cups cornmeal
1 tablespoon grated orange zest
2 teaspoons honey
¾ cup maple syrup

Place 2½ cups of the orange juice and the water in a saucepan. Bring to a boil; reduce the heat and gradually add the cornmeal while stirring. Add the orange zest and honey. Cook, stirring, until the mixture is very thick, about 10 minutes. Spread in a nonstick 8 × 8-inch baking dish. Cover with plastic wrap and chill overnight.

In the morning, remove the polenta from the pan and slice it in half, and then slice ½-inch-thick pieces crosswise. You should end up with about 24 slices. Brown just what you need for breakfast on a dry, nonstick griddle. Refrigerate the remainder in plastic wrap and use in a few days, or freeze for later use.

Combine the remaining ¼ cup orange juice with the maple syrup. Heat briefly. Serve over the browned polenta slices.

Cornmeal Cake

SERVINGS: 4 TO 7
PREPARATION TIME: 5 MINUTES
COOKING TIME: 45 TO 50 MINUTES

Serve this with any of the fruit sauces in this chapter, or try it with one of your favorite salsas.

4¼ cups water	1½ cups coarse cornmeal or
½ teaspoon salt (optional)	polenta

Heat 2 cups of the water and the salt in a large saucepan until boiling furiously. Add the cornmeal to the remaining 2½ cups cold water. Mix and add to the boiling water, stirring constantly. Bring the mixture to a boil and stir until smooth and thick. Cover the pan. Lower the heat and continue cooking gently for 30 to 40 minutes, stirring occasionally.

Pour into an 8- or 9-inch square nonstick baking dish. Cool for 1 hour or longer and then reheat in a 300°F oven for 20 minutes. Cut into squares and serve.

Variations: Add ⅓ cup uncooked millet to the mixture after it thickens, just before covering and cooking for 30 to 40 minutes.

Add 1 cup frozen corn kernels about 10 minutes before the end of the final cooking time.

Breakfast Tortillas

SERVINGS: 6 TO 8
PREPARATION TIME: 10 MINUTES (NEED COOKED RICE)
COOKING TIME: 10 MINUTES

2 cups firmly packed spinach, washed and chopped	1 cup frozen corn kernels
	½ cup salsa
	6 to 8 whole-wheat or corn tortillas
2 cups cooked brown rice	

Place the spinach in a saucepan with only the water you washed it in still clinging to the leaves. (If you washed the spinach the night before, place the spinach in the saucepan and sprinkle a little water over the leaves.) Cook, stirring, until just wilted, about 2 minutes. Remove from the saucepan and drain well.

Place the brown rice, corn, and salsa in the saucepan. Cook, stirring, until heated through. Stir in the spinach. Spoon a line of this mixture down the center of each tortilla and roll.

McDougall's Breakfast Burritos

SERVINGS: 6 TO 8
PREPARATION TIME: 10 MINUTES
COOKING TIME: 10 MINUTES

¼ cup chopped scallion	1 tablespoon soy sauce
¼ cup chopped green bell pepper	¼ to ½ teaspoon ground turmeric
¼ cup water	Freshly ground pepper to taste
1 tablespoon diced pimiento	6 to 8 whole-wheat tortillas
1 tablespoon diced canned green chilies	Salsa for garnish
1 pound (2 cups) firm tofu, crumbled	

Sauté the scallion and green pepper in the water for 5 minutes. Add the pimiento and green chilies. Stir. Add the remaining ingredients. Cook, stirring, over medium heat for about 5 minutes. Spoon a line of this mixture down the center of a tortilla. Add salsa if desired. Roll.

Breads

Basic Cornbread

SERVINGS: MAKES ONE 8-INCH SQUARE LOAF
PREPARATION TIME: 20 MINUTES
COOKING TIME: 30 MINUTES

You can purchase oat flour, millet flour, and rice milk at a natural-foods store. If you have a flour mill, you can grind your own flours. The recipe for rice milk (if you choose to make your own) is on page 90.

2 cups cornmeal
½ cup whole-wheat flour
⅓ cup oat flour
⅓ cup millet flour
4 teaspoons baking powder
2 cups rice milk

4 tablespoons frozen apple juice concentrate, thawed
3 teaspoons Ener-G Egg Replacer, well beaten with 4 tablespoons water

Preheat the oven to 375°F.

Mix the cornmeal, flours, and baking powder together and set aside. Mix the remaining ingredients together and pour over the dry ingredients. Fold together briefly. Pour into a nonstick 8-inch square pan. Bake for 30 minutes, or until a toothpick inserted in the center comes out clean.

Applesauce Cornbread Loaf

SERVINGS: MAKES TWO 9 x 5-INCH LOAVES
PREPARATION TIME: 20 MINUTES
COOKING TIME: 1 HOUR

Serve with your favorite natural preserves.

4 cups cornmeal
2 cups whole-wheat pastry
    flour
¾ cup millet
1 teaspoon salt

1 tablespoon baking powder
1 cup applesauce
¾ cup honey
2 teaspoons rice vinegar
3 cups low-fat soy milk

Preheat the oven to 350°F.

Place the cornmeal, flour, millet, salt, and baking powder in a large mixing bowl. Stir to combine.

Place the applesauce, honey, vinegar, and soy milk in a blender or food processor. Blend. Pour the wet ingredients into the dry and mix well (approximately 2 minutes).

Pour the batter into two nonstick 9 × 5-inch loaf pans. Bake for 1 hour, or until a toothpick inserted in the center of the loaf comes out clean. If it does not, reduce the oven temperature to 300°F and continue to bake until done. Check every 10 minutes after the first hour.

Remove the pans from the oven and let cool for 10 minutes before turning the loaves out of the pans. Cool completely on a rack.

Variation: Substitute rice flour for whole-wheat flour, or use 1 cup rice flour and 1 cup whole-wheat pastry flour. Rice flour results in a heavier (more dense) bread which will not rise as high.

Whole-Wheat Banana Bread

SERVINGS: MAKES TWO 8 x 5-INCH LOAVES
PREPARATION TIME: 15 MINUTES
COOKING TIME: 45 TO 55 MINUTES

4 cups whole-wheat flour
2 tablespoons wheat germ
2 teaspoons baking soda
6 teaspoons Ener-G Egg
Replacer, well beaten with
8 tablespoons water
4 cups mashed ripe banana
(about 16 medium bananas)

1 cup honey
½ cup water or unsweetened
juice
2 teaspoons vanilla extract
2 cups chopped walnuts
2 cups raisins

Preheat the oven to 350°F.

In a large bowl, combine the flour, wheat germ, and baking soda. Set aside.

In a food processor, combine the Egg Replacer, banana, honey, water, and vanilla. (If you do not have a food processor, do this in batches in a blender.) Pour this mixture over the dry ingredients. Stir in the walnuts and raisins.

Mix well and pour into two 8 × 5-inch nonstick loaf pans. Bake for 45 to 55 minutes, or until a toothpick inserted in the center comes out clean. Let cool in the pan for 10 minutes, then loosen the sides with a spatula, invert, and remove from the pan. Cool completely on a rack.

Note: This bread freezes well.

Zucchini Bread

SERVINGS: ONE 8 x 4-INCH LOAF
PREPARATION TIME: 25 MINUTES
COOKING TIME: 1¼ HOURS

¼ cup mashed banana (about 1 medium banana)
1 cup grated fresh zucchini
¼ cup frozen grape juice concentrate, thawed
1 tablespoon fresh lemon juice
1 teaspoon vanilla extract
2 cups whole-wheat pastry flour
½ teaspoon baking soda
2 teaspoons baking powder
1 teaspoon grated lemon zest
2 teaspoons ground cinnamon
½ cup raisins

Preheat the oven to 350°F.

In a large bowl, combine the banana, zucchini, juices, and vanilla. Blend well. In a separate large bowl, combine the remaining ingredients. Pour the wet ingredients into the dry and mix thoroughly. Pour into a nonstick 8 x 4-inch loaf pan and bake for about 1¼ hours, or until a toothpick inserted in the center comes out clean. Let cool in the pan for 10 minutes, then loosen the sides gently with a spatula, invert, and remove from the pan. Cool completely on a rack.

Whole-Wheat Bagels

SERVINGS: MAKES 16 TO 18 BAGELS
PREPARATION TIME: 30 MINUTES, PLUS 20 MINUTES RISING TIME
COOKING TIME: 30 MINUTES

2 tablespoons active dry
yeast
1 tablespoon honey
2½ cups warm water
6 cups whole-wheat or
unbleached white flour
(see Note 1)

2 tablespoons sesame or
poppy seeds (optional)

In a large bowl, mix the yeast, honey, and water. Add 2 cups of the flour and beat with a whisk. Let rise for 10 minutes. Add 4 more cups of flour while turning out on a board. Knead for 10 minutes, or until the dough is soft but not sticky. Tear or cut off pieces to make rolls about 8 inches long and 1 inch thick. Dip one end in water and attach it to the other end to make bagel shapes. Let rise on a floured board for 5 to 10 minutes.

Fill a large pot two-thirds full of water, and bring to a boil. Place the bagels in the boiling water with a slotted spoon, risen side down, four at a time. Cover the pot and let the bagels boil for about 30 seconds on each side, using a slotted spoon to gently flip them over. Watch them rise!

Meanwhile, preheat the oven to 375°F.

Remove the bagels from the water and place them on a nonstick cookie sheet, ½ inch apart. When they are fairly dry, you can sprinkle them with sesame seeds or poppy seeds. Bake for 25 to 30 minutes, or until lightly browned. Remove from the oven and let the bagels cool on a rack.

Notes: 1. I use 3 cups unbleached and 3 cups whole-wheat flour, which yields a nice, light bagel.

2. You can add sautéed onions, caraway seeds, blueberries, or just about anything you can think of for flavor.

Oil-Free Stone-Ground Whole-Wheat Bread (Recipe for Hitachi Automatic Bread Machine)

SERVINGS: MAKES 1 LOAF
PREPARATION TIME: 20 MINUTES
COOKING TIME: 4 HOURS, 10 MINUTES

There are many different brands of automatic bread-making machines on the market. These machines all use the basic ingredients (flour, water, and yeast) and do the mixing, kneading, rising, and baking for you. All you have to do is pour in the ingredients, push a few buttons, and leave it alone for several hours. Most recipes that come with bread machines, however, use butter, oil, eggs, and dairy products. This recipe was developed for those of you who have bread machines and are looking for a healthy bread recipe.

3 cups whole-wheat flour	1½ cups water at 110°F
⅜ cup wheat gluten flour	4 teaspoons active dry yeast
2 heaping teaspoons salt	3 tablespoons honey

Mix the flour, gluten flour, and salt in a large bowl.

Pour the water into the bread machine's pan. (It is important to use a thermometer to ensure that the water is precisely 110°F.) Sprinkle the yeast into the water. Stir with a wooden spoon until the yeast is thoroughly dissolved. Add the honey. Stir with a wooden spoon until the honey is thoroughly dissolved. Add the flour mixture. Gently stir in each corner of the pan to mix thoroughly.

Place the pan in the bread machine. Set on Bread menu. Push Start and Lock buttons, choosing a medium or light crust setting.

Note: This recipe was developed by Marylyn Spomer for the Hitachi Home Bread Machine and sold to the Hitachi Corporation. Permission was granted by Mr. Bob Sisco of the Hitachi Corporation to print this recipe in this cookbook.

Oil-Free Stone-Ground Whole-Wheat Dinner Rolls: Prepare the dough as directed above, but set the machine on the Dough menu. When completed, remove the dough. Divide it into two equal parts and roll out to a 1-inch thickness with a rolling pin. Make twelve balls from each of the two equal parts, for a total of twenty-four. Place twelve balls on each of two nonstick baking sheets. Place the baking sheets on top of the oven or in another warm spot. Spray lightly with water, cover with a warm damp cloth, and let rise for 1 hour, or until doubled in size.

Preheat the oven to 350°F.

Bake for 13 to 15 minutes, or until golden brown, on the middle oven rack.

Sweet Bread: Prepare the dough as directed above, but increase the quantity of honey to 6 tablespoons.

Sweet Rolls: Set on the dough menu. When ready, divide the dough in half, roll out lengthwise. Spread Cinnamon Paste (below) all over the dough. Then down the center of the dough put raisins and ground nuts or, instead of raisins, dates can be used. Fold the dough over like a jelly roll and slice. Place the slices in a muffin tin (Teflon). Place on the stove or a warm spot, spray lightly with water, cover with a warm damp cloth. Let rise 1 hour. They will double in size. Bake at 350°F for 13 to 15 minutes or until golden brown. Place on the center rack in a conventional oven. Will freeze well.

Cinnamon Paste

This goes well with the recipe for Sweet Rolls.

6 tablespoons honey

3 heaping tablespoons ground cinnamon

Blend the honey and cinnamon thoroughly.

Muffins

Basic Corn Muffins

SERVINGS: MAKES 12 MUFFINS
PREPARATION TIME: 10 MINUTES
COOKING TIME: 15 MINUTES

Two 6-ounce cartons plain
  soy yogurt
⅔ cup water
2 teaspoons Ener-G Egg
  Replacer, well beaten
  with 4 tablespoons
  water

2 cups cornmeal
2 teaspoons baking
  powder
1 teaspoon baking soda
½ teaspoon salt

Preheat the oven to 475°F.

Blend the yogurt, water, and Egg Replacer mixture thoroughly. Mix the remaining ingredients together and add to the wet ingredients. Spoon the batter into twelve nonstick muffin cups and bake for 15 minutes, or until lightly browned.

Apple–Oat Bran Muffins

SERVINGS: MAKES 12 MUFFINS
PREPARATION TIME: 15 MINUTES
COOKING TIME: 20 MINUTES

1 cup oat flour
¾ cup oat bran
½ teaspoon baking soda
¼ teaspoon ground nutmeg
¼ cup honey
¼ cup unsulphured molasses
2 teaspoons Ener-G Egg Replacer, mixed with 4 tablespoons water and beaten until frothy
¾ cup low-fat vanilla soy milk

¼ cup any unsweetened fruit juice
1 medium apple, cored, skinned, and chopped
¼ cup raisins, chopped dried dates, or chopped dried pineapple
½ teaspoon grated orange zest

Preheat the oven to 400°F.

Mix the flour, oat bran, baking soda, and nutmeg in a large bowl. In a separate bowl, combine the remaining ingredients. Pour the wet mixture into the dry and stir until mixed. Spoon the batter into twelve nonstick muffin cups. Bake for 20 minutes, or until lightly browned.

Easy Muffins: Three Variations

SERVINGS: MAKES 18 MUFFINS (PER VARIATION)
PREPARATION TIME: 10 MINUTES
COOKING TIME: 30 MINUTES

1. OAT BRAN MUFFINS

2 cups whole-wheat pastry flour
2 cups oat bran
4 teaspoons baking powder
½ cup raisins (optional)
½ cup chopped walnuts (optional)

1 teaspoon ground cinnamon (optional)
2 cups unsweetened apple juice

2. CORNBREAD MUFFINS

2 cups cornmeal
2 cups oat bran
4 teaspoons baking powder

2 cups unsweetened apple juice

3. BANANA MUFFINS

2 cups whole-wheat flour
2 cups oat bran
4 teaspoons baking powder
½ cup raisins (optional)

2 cups mashed ripe banana (3 to 4 bananas)
½ cup unsweetened apple juice

Preheat the oven to 350°F.

Sift the dry ingredients together. Add the optional ingredients if using. Add the wet ingredients and stir until just mixed. Spoon the batter into eighteen nonstick muffin cups and bake for 30 minutes, or until lightly browned.

Fruity Carrot-Bran Muffins

SERVINGS: MAKES 15 MUFFINS
PREPARATION TIME: 15 MINUTES
COOKING TIME: 30 TO 35 MINUTES

2½ cups whole-wheat flour
½ cup wheat bran
2 teaspoons baking powder
½ teaspoon baking soda
½ cup chopped walnuts
(optional)
½ cup chopped dried
apricots
¼ cup raisins

3 teaspoons Ener-G Egg
Replacer, mixed with 6
tablespoons water and
beaten until foamy
½ cup low-fat soy milk
1 cup grated carrot
¾ cup fresh-squeezed orange
juice
½ cup honey

Preheat the oven to 350°F.

In a large mixing bowl, combine the flour, bran, baking powder, and baking soda. Add the nuts, apricots, and raisins to the dry ingredients, mixing well to prevent large lumps. Pour the Egg Replacer mixture into a blender. Add the soy milk, carrot, and orange juice. Process briefly. Pour the wet ingredients into the dry ingredients; add the honey. Mix just until moistened. Spoon the batter into fifteen nonstick muffin cups. Bake for 30 to 35 minutes, or until lightly browned.

Zucchini Muffins

SERVINGS: MAKES 18 MUFFINS
PREPARATION TIME: 20 MINUTES
COOKING TIME: 20 MINUTES

These are my favorite muffins. They are easy to make perfect the first time you try.

3 cups oat bran
1 cup boiling water
3 teaspoons Ener-G Egg Replacer, beaten with 4 tablespoons water until frothy
¾ cup honey
2 cups low-fat soy milk

2 cups grated zucchini
2 cups whole-wheat pastry flour
2½ teaspoons baking soda
½ teaspoon ground cinnamon
½ teaspoon ground cloves

Preheat the oven to 375°F.

Place the oat bran in a large mixing bowl. Add the boiling water and stir to mix. Set aside.

Combine the Egg Replacer mixture with the honey and soy milk. Pour into the oat-bran mixture and beat with an electric beater until no lumps remain. Stir in the grated zucchini. Add the remaining ingredients and stir until well mixed.

Spoon the batter into eighteen nonstick muffin cups. Bake for 20 minutes, or until lightly browned.

Variations: Substitute any of the following for the grated zucchini: 2 cups grated apple; 2 cups blueberries; 2 cups *well-drained* crushed pineapple; 1½ cups raisins.

CHAPTER 4

DIPS, SANDWICH SPREADS, AND ACCOMPANIMENTS

What do you put on your sandwich if you're not going to use meat and cheese? The vegetarian options are endless once you consider the possibilities. Roasted Garlic Spread, Millet Butter, Curried Bean Spread, Eggplant Spread, Tofu Cream Cheese, Broccomole, and Sandwich Cheese use ingredients from all corners of the plant kingdom. The color, flavor, texture, and aroma of these spreads will leave you asking, "How could I have been content with brown and yellow spreads that tasted of fat and salt (lunch meats and cheeses) for all those years?"

These spreads can also be used as dips. Make Oven-Baked Tortilla Chips or Garlic-Pita Wedges to dip into these delicious spreads and dips. An assortment of raw vegetables makes an excellent hors d'oeurve tray to serve at a dinner party. You will likely want to keep a supply of your favorite dips and spreads handy in the refrigerator to add extra flavor to almost any of your favorite snacks and dishes. This is simply a way to invigorate the taste of the simplest foods, like a humble baked potato.

Several of the recipes, such as Tofu Cream Cheese, Tofu "Egg" Salad, and Tofu Artichoke Spread, as the names imply, are made primarily of tofu, which is low in fiber and over 50 percent fat.

Please consider the richness of these recipes when you're planning your menu for the sake of your health and appearance.

Broccomole

SERVINGS: MAKES 2 CUPS
PREPARATION TIME: 10 MINUTES (NEED COOKED BROCCOLI)
CHILLING TIME: 1 TO 2 HOURS

Serve this with burritos or tostados, or use as an appetizer with chips and salsa.

1½ cups cooked broccoli stems, tough outer layers peeled off	⅛ teaspoon garlic powder
	½ tomato, diced
	1 scallion, sliced
1½ tablespoons fresh-squeezed lemon juice	1 canned green chili, chopped
¼ teaspoon ground cumin	

In a food processor, blend the broccoli stems with the lemon juice, cumin, and garlic powder until completely smooth. Add the remaining ingredients and mix well by hand, but do not blend. Chill before serving for best flavor.

Roasted Garlic Spread

SERVINGS: VARIABLE
PREPARATION TIME: 5 MINUTES
COOKING TIME: 1 TO 1¼ HOURS

Spread on toast or crackers for a delicious treat.

1 head garlic (try elephant garlic)

Preheat the oven to 300°F.

Remove the loose, papery outer skin from the garlic. Put the whole head, root-end down, in a shallow baking dish. Roast for 1 to 1¼ hours, or until the garlic is soft. Cool until it is easy to handle.

Squeeze the soft garlic out of the skin.

Variation: Mix the roasted garlic with 3 cups cooked white beans. Process in a blender or food processor until smooth. Add ¼ teaspoon crushed red pepper flakes for a spicier spread.

Garbanzo Guacamole

SERVINGS: MAKES 2 CUPS
PREPARATION TIME: 15 MINUTES
CHILLING TIME: 2 TO 4 HOURS

This is a lower-fat version of the traditional guacamole. Because of the small amount of avocado used, however, it still contains some fat. To reduce the amount of fat, eliminate the avocado. The recipe will still be delicious. Serve with oil-free tortilla chips or fresh vegetables.

One 15-ounce can garbanzo beans, rinsed and drained
1 tablespoon fresh lemon juice
1 clove garlic, crushed
1 medium onion, chopped
½ small avocado, peeled and chopped (optional)
1 medium tomato, chopped
4 scallions, thinly sliced
1 tablespoon canned chopped green chilies

Place the garbanzo beans in a food processor or blender. Add the lemon juice and garlic. Process briefly, until the garbanzos are slightly chopped. Add the onion and the avocado, if desired. Process again until the mixture is chunky. Place the mixture in a bowl and add the remaining ingredients. Mix well. Cover and chill before serving.

Cucumber Dip

SERVINGS: MAKES 1½ CUPS
PREPARATION TIME: 10 MINUTES

This is a wonderful dip for bread or raw vegetables!

1 cucumber
1 cup plain soy yogurt
3 to 4 cloves garlic, crushed

¼ teaspoon white pepper, or to taste

Peel the cucumber and cut it in half lengthwise. Scoop out and discard the seeds; coarsely chop the cucumber. Place it in a food processor and chop very fine. (This may also be done with a hand grater.) Remove from the food processor and place in a very fine strainer. Press out as much water as possible. Return to the food processor (or place in a blender). Add the remaining ingredients and process until fairly smooth. Add more garlic and/or white pepper to taste. Refrigerate for several hours before using, for best flavor.

Tempeh Pâté

SERVINGS: 8
PREPARATION TIME: 15 MINUTES
COOKING TIME: 15 MINUTES
CHILLING TIME: 1 TO 2 HOURS

Serve on crackers or as a sandwich spread. For tempeh balls, form the pâté into 1-inch balls and bake at 350°F for 10 to 15 minutes. This is a high-fat, high-salt recipe to be used sparingly by healthy people.

One 8-ounce package five-
  grain tempeh
2 tablespoons soy sauce
3 tablespoons tofu
  mayonnaise

¼ cup chopped celery
2 tablespoons minced
  scallion
½ teaspoon dried dill

Steam the tempeh for 10 to 15 minutes. Mash the tempeh with the soy sauce and tofu mayonnaise in a bowl. Sauté the celery and scallion in a small amount of water for a few minutes. Add to the tempeh and mix well. Add the dill. Mix again and chill.

Millet Butter

SERVINGS: MAKES 2½ CUPS
PREPARATION TIME: 15 MINUTES
COOKING TIME: 40 MINUTES

Try this on muffins or toast.

⅓ cup millet
2½ cups water
¼ cup minced carrot
1 teaspoon agar-agar
    powder or 1 tablespoon
    agar-agar flakes (see Note)

¼ cup raw cashews
½ teaspoon salt (optional)

Place the millet in a saucepan with 1 cup of the water. Cover and cook over low heat for about 40 minutes, or until the liquid is absorbed.

Meanwhile, cook the carrot and agar-agar in the remaining 1½ cups water for 10 minutes, stirring occasionally. Remove from the heat. Pour half of this mixture into a blender and add the cooked millet, the cashews, and the salt. Blend until very smooth. Add the remaining carrot mixture and blend again. Pour into a container with a tight-fitting lid, but do not cover until cooled slightly. Refrigerate before serving.

Note: You can substitute 2 tablespoons of Emes gelatin for the agar-agar. See page 72 for discussions of both Emes gelatin and agar-agar.

Indian Lentil Sandwich Spread

SERVINGS: MAKES 1 CUP
PREPARATION TIME: 5 MINUTES (NEED COOKED LENTILS)
COOKING TIME: 5 MINUTES
CHILLING TIME: 1 HOUR

Use as a sandwich spread or stuff into pita "pockets."

1 cup cooked lentils	½ teaspoon ground turmeric
4 cloves garlic, pressed	½ teaspoon chili powder
2 teaspoons ground coriander	½ teaspoon ground ginger
1 teaspoon ground cumin	

Combine all of the ingredients in a small saucepan. Cook gently over low heat, stirring occasionally, for 5 minutes, to allow the flavors to blend. Chill for 1 hour.

Curried Bean Sandwich Spread

SERVINGS: MAKES 4 CUPS
PREPARATION TIME: 20 MINUTES (NEED COOKED BEANS)
COOKING TIME: 15 MINUTES
CHILLING TIME: 1 HOUR

Use as a spread on sandwiches or stuff into pita bread.

¾ cup water	1 to 2 cloves garlic, minced
1 onion, finely chopped	2½ teaspoons curry powder
1 cup diced celery	½ teaspoon ground cumin
1 green bell pepper, diced	1 tablespoon soy sauce
½ cup diced carrot	3 cups cooked white beans

Place the water in a saucepan and add all of the vegetables and the garlic. Cook, stirring occasionally, for 15 minutes. Stir in the curry powder, cumin, and soy sauce, and mix well. Remove from the heat. Add the beans; mix well. Place the mixture in a food processor or blender and process briefly until chopped but not pureed. Chill.

Eggplant Spread

SERVINGS: MAKES 1 CUP
PREPARATION TIME: 1 HOUR 10 MINUTES
COOKING TIME: 10 MINUTES
CHILLING TIME: 1 TO 2 HOURS

Try this spicy spread on sandwiches or as a dip.

1 eggplant (1 to 1½ pounds)
2 tablespoons minced fresh parsley
2 tablespoons minced fresh cilantro
1 teaspoon ground cumin

1 teaspoon ground coriander
½ teaspoon garlic powder
¼ teaspoon salt (optional)
Dash or two Tabasco

Preheat the oven to 350°F.

Cut the stem off the eggplant and prick it all over with a fork. Place it directly on the oven rack and bake for about 1 hour, or until the eggplant is soft and the skin is wrinkled. Remove from the oven and allow to cool.

When it is cool enough to handle, peel and chop. Place in a blender or food processor with the parsley and cilantro. Process until smooth. Place in a saucepan and add the remaining ingredients. Cook, stirring, until the mixture thickens slightly, about 10 minutes. Chill.

Tofu Cream Cheese

SERVINGS: MAKES 1 CUP
PREPARATION TIME: 15 MINUTES
COOKING TIME: 1 MINUTE   CHILLING TIME: 1 TO 2 HOURS

Makes a very rich, delicious sandwich spread.

½ pound firm tofu
2 tablespoons fresh lemon
  juice
½ teaspoon onion powder
½ teaspoon garlic powder
2 tablespoons chopped green
  bell pepper

2 tablespoons chopped
  scallion
2 tablespoons chopped
  celery
2 tablespoons chopped
  radish

Place the tofu in a saucepan with water to cover and bring to a boil. Boil for 1 minute. Drain. Place the tofu in a clean linen napkin or a double thickness of cheesecloth and draw the ends together to form a sack. Twist gently, squeezing out all the water.

Place the tofu in a food processor or blender with the lemon juice, onion powder, and garlic powder. Process until smooth. Pour into a covered container, mix in the chopped vegetables, and chill for an hour or two before serving.

Tofu Artichoke Spread

SERVINGS: MAKES 3 CUPS
PREPARATION TIME: 15 MINUTES
CHILLING TIME: 1 TO 2 HOURS

This is an interesting and delicious way to use artichokes.

One 14-ounce can water-
  packed artichoke hearts
  or 1 package frozen
  artichoke hearts, thawed
1 pound tofu, drained

1 small onion, minced
4 tablespoons oil-free
  Italian dressing
½ teaspoon garlic powder
  Dash or two Tabasco

Place the artichoke hearts in a blender or food processor and process until smooth. Place the tofu in a bowl and mash with a potato masher. Add the blended artichoke hearts and the remaining ingredients. Mix well and chill for an hour or two.

Tofu "Egg" Salad

SERVINGS: MAKES 2 CUPS
PREPARATION TIME: 10 MINUTES   CHILLING TIME: 1 HOUR

Serve as a spread on bread or stuff into pita bread.

1 pound firm tofu, drained and crumbled
¼ cup fat-free mayonnaise (optional; see Note)
2 tablespoons prepared mustard
1 tablespoon soy sauce
½ teaspoon ground turmeric
3 to 4 scallions, finely chopped
¼ cup minced celery
⅛ cup pickle relish (optional)

Place the tofu in a bowl and mash with a potato masher. Add the mayonnaise (if desired), mustard, soy sauce, and turmeric. Mix well until the tofu takes on a bright yellow color. Stir in the scallions, celery, and relish, if desired. Chill 1 hour or more before serving.

Note: Weight Watchers makes a mayonnaise that is fat free; it contains no oil and no eggs.

Tofu "Chicken" Salad

SERVINGS: MAKES ABOUT 2 CUPS
PREPARATION TIME: 20 MINUTES
CHILLING TIME: 2 TO 3 HOURS

This is rich in contrast to other McDougall recipes, but much healthier than chicken or egg salad; for example—lower in fat and cholesterol free. Serve on whole-wheat bread with the garnishes of your choice, or stuff into pita bread and garnish with lettuce leaves and sliced fresh mushrooms.

1 pound tofu, drained
¼ cup finely chopped red onion
¼ cup finely chopped celery
¼ cup finely chopped green bell pepper
¼ cup finely chopped red bell pepper
2 tablespoons oil-free Italian dressing
1 tablespoon low-sodium soy sauce
1 teaspoon fresh lemon juice
¼ teaspoon ground turmeric
¼ teaspoon garlic powder
Dash cayenne pepper

Crumble the tofu into a bowl and mash with a potato masher. Add the remaining ingredients and mix well. Refrigerate for a few hours to allow the flavors to blend.

Mockzarella Cheese

SERVINGS: MAKES 3 CUPS
PREPARATION TIME: 20 MINUTES
COOKING TIME: 5 MINUTES
CHILLING TIME: 2 HOURS OR MORE

1½ cups raw cashews, rinsed
2 cups water
¼ cup raw sesame seeds
1 small onion, chopped
1 teaspoon crushed fresh garlic
2 tablespoons fresh lemon juice

¼ cup pimientos	2 teaspoons arrowroot
3 teaspoons active dry	powder
yeast	1 teaspoon salt

Put the cashews in a blender or food processor with 1½ cups of the water. Process until smooth and creamy. Add the sesame seeds, onion, garlic, and lemon juice, plus the remaining ½ cup water, and process until smooth. Add the remaining ingredients and process again until smooth.

Pour the mixture into a saucepan. Cook over low heat, stirring constantly, until the mixture thickens—about 5 minutes.

Spoon into a covered container. Refrigerate for at least 2 hours before serving.

Sandwich Cheese

SERVINGS: MAKES 1½ CUPS
PREPARATION TIME: 10 MINUTES
COOKING TIME: 5 MINUTES   CHILLING TIME: 1 HOUR

This is an excellent spread for sandwiches, grilled or otherwise.

1 cup water	2 tablespoons raw sesame
1 tablespoon agar-agar	seeds
flakes (see Note, page 119)	3 tablespoons active dry
3 tablespoons pimientos	yeast
3 tablespoons fresh lemon	½ teaspoon salt (optional)
juice	½ teaspoon onion powder
2 tablespoons raw cashews	⅛ teaspoon garlic powder

Place the water and agar-agar in a small saucepan and bring to a boil. Boil until clear, about 5 minutes. Place all of the remaining ingredients in a blender; add the hot liquid. Blend first on low, then on high (otherwise hot liquid may overflow). While the mixture is still in the blender, add a few extra chopped pimientos or green chilies (as desired). Pulse the blender on and off just to mix.

Pour into a container with a tight-fitting lid. Do this immediately, as the cheese sets very fast. Chill in the refrigerator for 1 hour or longer.

Oven-Baked Tortilla Chips

SERVINGS: MAKES 96 CHIPS
PREPARATION TIME: 5 MINUTES
COOKING TIME: 5 TO 7 MINUTES

These are a delicious substitute for the greasy corn chips you used to dip in salsas and bean dips. John's father takes a bag of these chips along with him whenever he goes out to eat in a Mexican restaurant. There are some commercially made oil-free corn chips available in some parts of the country (see acceptable product list, pages 42–69).

12 soft corn tortillas

Preheat the oven to 450°F.
 Cut each tortilla into eight wedges. Lay them on a dry baking sheet in a single layer. Bake for 5 to 7 minutes, or until crisp. Watch them carefully so they don't burn. Store in an airtight container.

Easy Nonfat Garlic Bread

SERVINGS: 12
PREPARATION TIME: 15 MINUTES
COOKING TIME: 5 MINUTES

1 cup oil-free Italian dressing
1 teaspoon paprika
5 cloves garlic (or more to taste)

1 loaf whole-wheat French bread
Parsley flakes (optional)

Preheat the broiler.
 Place the dressing, paprika, and garlic in a blender and process until well blended. Brush this mixture on the bread and sprinkle with parsley, if desired.

Broil until the bread turns a light golden brown. Watch carefully to make sure it doesn't burn.

Note: The garlic mixture will stay fresh for several weeks in the refrigerator if stored in a covered container.

Garlic Pita Wedges

SERVINGS: MAKES 32 WEDGES
PREPARATION TIME: 20 MINUTES
COOKING TIME: 15 MINUTES

½ cup oil-free Italian
 dressing
2 to 3 cloves garlic
¼ teaspoon paprika

4 whole-wheat pita breads,
 split into 8 circles
Finely chopped fresh
 parsley (optional)

Preheat the oven to 350°F.

Place the dressing, garlic, and paprika in a blender jar. Process until smooth. Transfer to a bowl.

Cut each pita circle into four wedges. Generously brush some of the garlic mixture on the inside of each wedge. Place the wedges in a single layer on a dry baking sheet, brushed sides up. Sprinkle with chopped parsley, if desired. Bake for about 15 minutes, or until browned.

Wheat-Free "Bread Crumbs"

SERVINGS: MAKES 3 CUPS
PREPARATION TIME: 5 MINUTES   COOKING TIME: 30 MINUTES

Millet may be used in place of bread crumbs in recipes like Stuffed Zucchini, Stuffed Mushroom Caps, or Carrot Loaf. The ratio of water to millet should be slightly less than three to one for the millet to be crumbly. Use the same amount of millet as you would bread crumbs called for in a recipe. People that have an allergy to wheat will find these an excellent substitute.

1 cup millet   2⅞ cups water

Place the millet in a saucepan with the water. Bring to a boil, then reduce the heat and simmer, partly covered, for 30 minutes. Fluff the millet with a fork before using. Extra millet may be stored in the refrigerator for several days or frozen for use later.

Bread-Crumb Mixtures

SERVINGS: MAKES 3½ CUPS
PREPARATION TIME: 5 TO 10 MINUTES
COOKING TIME: 1 TO 2 MINUTES OR NONE

Use these mixtures in any recipe calling for bread crumbs to give added flavor. Or sprinkle on top of various casseroles, such as Macaroni and Cabbage, Layered Vegetable Casserole, or Potato Kugel, before final baking.

CHEESY SOURDOUGH BREAD CRUMBS

**4 slices whole-wheat
  sourdough bread
1 to 2 tablespoons grated soy
  Parmesan cheese**

**1 tablespoon minced
  fresh parsley**

Break up the bread slices and process in a food processor or blender until finely chopped. Add the remaining ingredients and mix well. Store, covered, in the refrigerator.

HERBED BREAD CRUMBS

4 slices whole-wheat bread	1 tablespoon minced fresh parsley
2 to 3 cloves garlic, crushed	

Break up the bread slices and process in a blender or food processor until finely chopped. Add the garlic; mix well. Transfer to a nonstick frying pan and cook over medium-low heat for 1 to 2 minutes, stirring constantly so the crumbs don't burn. Add the parsley, mix well, and store, covered, in the refrigerator.

Croutons

SERVINGS: MAKES ABOUT 3 CUPS
PREPARATION TIME: 15 MINUTES
COOKING TIME: 30 TO 45 MINUTES

Sprinkle these on top of salads or stir into soups. They also may be eaten as a crispy snack food.

1 loaf oil-free whole-wheat   ⅔ cup tomato juice
  bread   ⅛ cup onion powder

Flavoring Alternatives

ITALIAN FLAVOR

1½ tablespoons dried basil   1 teaspoon dried oregano
1 tablespoon garlic powder   ½ teaspoon dried thyme

SPANISH FLAVOR

1 tablespoon garlic powder   ½ tablespoon ground cumin
1 tablespoon chili powder   ½ tablespoon paprika

DILL FLAVOR

1½ tablespoons dried dill   1 teaspoon ground coriander
½ tablespoon garlic powder

Preheat the oven to 350°F.

Cut the bread into cubes and place them in a large bowl. Add the tomato juice and onion powder. Toss well to mix. Add spices from the list above, if desired. Place the bread cubes on nonstick baking sheets. Bake for 30 to 45 minutes, stirring every 15 minutes, watching carefully to make sure they don't burn. They should be lightly browned and crispy.

CHAPTER 5

SOUPS, STEWS, AND CHILIS

Served with your favorite bread, a baked potato, or rice, soups, stews, and chilis make a delicious one-pot meal. A complimentary but not essential addition to the meal might be a green salad. This chapter might stretch your comfort zone by introducing you to many recipes with exotic ingredients. To ease into this adventure start with Vegetable Chowder, Cream of Broccoli Soup, and Hearty Brown Stew. Once you have discovered what an enjoyable dining experience these recipes provide, make Green Gnocchi Soup, Sopa Seca, Black Bean Soup with Cilantro and Orange, Spicy Yam Stew, Squash and Tomato Stew, Three-Bean Chili, Texas Crude, or Extra-Spicy Lentil Chili.

Consider carefully the base of the soup, stew, or chili when choosing a recipe. Common ingredients include beans, pasta, potatoes, rice, and corn. Choose flavoring ingredients carefully—the spices you add will ultimately make the meal.

Soups

Hearty Vegetable Broth

SERVINGS: MAKES ABOUT 6 QUARTS
PREPARATION TIME: 15 MINUTES
COOKING TIME: 3 TO 4 HOURS

This broth is more concentrated in flavor and contains more salt than the Light Vegetable Broth on the next page. Use in any recipe calling for vegetable broth, or use in place of water in other soup recipes for extra flavor.

5 quarts water
2 large onions, peeled and quartered
4 to 5 cloves garlic, peeled
4 stalks celery, thickly sliced
4 large carrots, scrubbed and thickly sliced
2 large potatoes, scrubbed and coarsely chopped

2 leeks, white parts only, washed and thickly sliced
Several large sprigs fresh parsley
2 bay leaves
10 whole peppercorns
4 tablespoons soy sauce

Place all of the ingredients in a large soup pot. Bring to a boil, reduce the heat, cover, and simmer over low heat for 3 to 4 hours. Strain the broth and discard the vegetables.

Freeze in 1- to 2-cup containers for use in recipes calling for vegetable stock or broth.

Light Vegetable Broth

SERVINGS: MAKES ABOUT 8 QUARTS
PREPARATION TIME: 30 MINUTES
COOKING TIME: 3 TO 4 HOURS

6½ quarts water
2 cups white wine or unsweetened apple juice
6 stalks celery, thickly sliced
6 carrots, scrubbed and coarsely chopped
2 large potatoes, scrubbed and coarsely chopped
3 medium zucchini, thickly sliced
2 large onions, chopped
1 leek, white part only, cleaned and thickly sliced
5 to 6 cloves garlic, crushed
½ pound mushrooms, cleaned and left whole
10 whole peppercorns
Several large sprigs fresh parsley
Several large sprigs fresh thyme
2 bay leaves

Place all of the ingredients in a large soup pot. Bring to a boil, reduce the heat, cover, and simmer over low heat for 3 to 4 hours. Strain the broth and discard the vegetables.

Freeze in 1- to 2-cup containers for use in recipes calling for vegetable stock or broth.

Use this in any recipe calling for vegetable broth. It is low in sodium but still rich in flavor.

Miso Soup

SERVINGS: 4
PREPARATION TIME: 10 MINUTES
COOKING TIME: 5 MINUTES

1 quart water	¼ cup chopped scallion
¼ cup mellow white miso	½ cup diced firm tofu
1 to 2 tablespoons soy sauce	

Place the water in a saucepan and bring to a boil. Place the miso in a small bowl. Add about ½ cup of the boiling water to the miso and mix well. Pour into the saucepan. Add 1 tablespoon of soy sauce, the scallion, and the tofu. Heat for 1 to 2 minutes. Taste and add additional soy sauce, if necessary. Stir often while serving to make sure the vegetables and tofu are well distributed.

Borscht

SERVINGS: 8
PREPARATION TIME: 30 MINUTES
COOKING TIME: 45 MINUTES

6 cups water	¼ cup chopped fresh parsley
4 cups shredded red cabbage	2 tablespoons honey
1 cup peeled julienned beets	2 teaspoons chopped fresh dill
1 onion, chopped	
2 cloves garlic, crushed	1 teaspoon paprika
2 large potatoes, peeled and chopped	Freshly ground pepper to taste
¼ cup red-wine vinegar	Fresh dill for garnish

Place all of the ingredients in a large soup pot, except the dill for garnish. Bring to a boil, cover, reduce the heat, and cook over medium heat for 45 minutes. Garnish with fresh dill.

Chunky Gazpacho

SERVINGS: 10
PREPARATION TIME: 20 TO 40 MINUTES
CHILLING TIME: 3 TO 4 HOURS

4 cups tomato juice
2 cups peeled, seeded, and chopped tomatoes (see Note)
1 cup chopped cucumber
½ cup chopped red onion
½ cup chopped celery
½ cup thawed frozen or fresh corn kernels
½ cup chopped green bell pepper
¼ cup chopped scallion

¼ cup chopped zucchini
¼ cup chopped mild green chilies
¼ cup chopped fresh parsley
¼ cup chopped fresh cilantro (optional)
1 to 2 cloves garlic, minced
2 tablespoons red-wine vinegar
2 tablespoons fresh lime juice

Combine all of the ingredients in a large bowl. Cover and chill for 3 to 4 hours before serving.

Note: To peel tomatoes, dip briefly in boiling water, until the skins loosen, then just slip the skins off.

The ingredients may be prepared in a food processor. This is a great time saver.

Variation: This may also be prepared by pureeing half of the ingredients in a food processor or blender and leaving the remaining ingredients finely chopped.

Vichyssoise

SERVINGS: 6 TO 8
PREPARATION TIME: 25 MINUTES
COOKING TIME: 1 HOUR
CHILLING TIME: 2 TO 4 HOURS

3 cups peeled and chunked potatoes
1½ cups chopped onion
½ cup sliced leek
5 cups water
⅛ teaspoon freshly ground white pepper

1 tablespoon soy sauce
1 cup low-fat soy milk
Freshly ground black pepper to taste
Chopped scallions or chives for garnish

Place the vegetables, water, white pepper, and soy sauce in a large pot. Simmer over medium heat until the potatoes are very soft, about 1 hour. Blend until smooth. Stir in the soy milk and fresh pepper. Chill for 2 to 4 hours. Garnish with chopped scallions or chives.

Potato-Leek Soup

SERVINGS: 4 TO 6
PREPARATION TIME: 20 MINUTES
COOKING TIME: 30 TO 40 MINUTES

4 cups peeled and chunked potatoes
4 cups water
2 leeks, white parts only, washed well and sliced
½ teaspoon onion powder
¼ teaspoon garlic powder

⅛ teaspoon freshly ground white pepper
¼ teaspoon dried dill (optional)
½ cup chopped scallion (optional)

Place the potatoes, water, and leeks in a medium-sized soup pot. Bring to a boil, reduce the heat, cover, and cook until the potatoes are tender, about 30 minutes. Transfer to a blender or food processor and process until smooth and creamy. Or transfer only half of the soup to a blender or processor and blend until smooth and creamy. Return to the pan and stir to mix. This will yield a creamy soup with chunks of vegetables.

Add the remaining ingredients. Heat through. (If you are using the optional ingredients, cook over very low heat for 10 minutes.) Serve.

Potato-Corn Chowder

SERVINGS: 8
PREPARATION TIME: 20 MINUTES
COOKING TIME: 45 MINUTES

2 onions, chopped
1½ cups chopped celery
6½ cups water
6 potatoes, peeled and chopped
4 cups frozen corn kernels
1 teaspoon dried marjoram
½ teaspoon dried thyme
½ teaspoon dried oregano
¼ teaspoon dried basil
¼ teaspoon dried rosemary
¼ teaspoon dried savory
1 cup low-fat soy milk
Chopped fresh parsley or basil for garnish (optional)

Place the onion and celery in a large soup pot with ½ cup of the water. Sauté, stirring occasionally, until tender, about 10 minutes. Add the remaining ingredients except the soy milk and fresh herbs. Cover and cook over medium heat until the potatoes are tender, about 30 minutes.

Remove about 1 cup of the soup and place in a blender or food processor. Puree and return to the soup pot. Add the soy milk. Stir well and heat through. Garnish with some chopped fresh parsley or basil before serving, if desired.

Cream of Broccoli Soup

SERVINGS: 4 TO 6
PREPARATION TIME: 20 MINUTES
COOKING TIME: 50 MINUTES

2 small leeks, washed and
sliced
2 cloves garlic, minced
⅓ cup water
4 medium red potatoes,
peeled and chopped
3 cups water
2 medium stalks broccoli,
one chopped and one cut
into small florets

2 cups cashew milk (page 91)
½ teaspoon dried thyme
1 bay leaf
Freshly ground pepper to
taste

Sauté the leek and garlic in the ⅓ cup water for 5 minutes. Add the remaining ingredients except the broccoli florets. Cover and cook over medium heat for 40 minutes, or until the potatoes are tender.

Remove the bay leaf. Blend the mixture, in batches, in a blender or food processor until smooth and creamy. Return to the pan and keep warm.

Meanwhile, place the broccoli florets in another saucepan with water to cover. Cover and cook over medium heat for 5 minutes. Drain. Add to the soup mixture. Season with freshly ground pepper to taste.

Variation: You may substitute cauliflower for broccoli in this recipe with delicious results!

Curried Broccoli Soup

SERVINGS: 6
PREPARATION TIME: 25 MINUTES
COOKING TIME: 25 MINUTES

1 medium onion,
chopped
1 clove garlic, pressed
4¼ cups water
1 large bunch broccoli,
chopped (see Note)

1 large green apple,
chopped
2 tablespoons soy sauce
2 to 3 teaspoons curry powder
One 8.45-ounce container
low-fat soy milk

Place the onion and garlic in a large pan with ¼ cup of the water. Cook, stirring, for several minutes to soften. Add the remaining 4 cups of water, the broccoli, apple, soy sauce, and curry powder. Cover and cook over low heat for 20 minutes.

Remove from the heat and puree in batches in a blender or food processor. Return to the pan. Stir in the soy milk. Heat through. Serve at once.

Note: Do not use the tough lower stalks of the broccoli for this soup. Use only the florets and tender upper stalks.

Potato-Cauliflower Soup

SERVINGS: 8 TO 10
PREPARATION TIME: 40 MINUTES
COOKING TIME: 45 MINUTES

2 large onions, chopped
1 medium head cauliflower, chopped
5 cups peeled and chopped potatoes
8 cups water
2 teaspoons dried dill

2 bay leaves
2 tablespoons soy sauce
Freshly ground pepper to taste
Chopped fresh parsley for garnish

Place the onions, cauliflower, and potatoes in a large pot with the water. Bring to a boil. Reduce the heat, add the dill, cover, and cook over medium heat until the potato and cauliflower are tender, about 30 minutes.

Remove from the heat and puree in batches in a blender or food processor. Return to the soup pot. Add the bay leaves, soy sauce, and pepper. Cook over low heat for 15 minutes to allow the flavors to blend. Remove the bay leaves and garnish with chopped fresh parsley before serving.

Zucchini Soup

SERVINGS: 6
PREPARATION TIME: 15 MINUTES   COOKING TIME: 15 MINUTES

A smooth, creamy green soup.

6 medium zucchini, chopped
5 cups water
1 small onion, chopped
2 cloves garlic
4 bay leaves

3 tablespoons vegetable seasoning/broth mix
½ cup soy milk or ¼ cup soy milk powder
Dash smoke flavoring (optional)

Place the zucchini, water, onion, garlic, and bay leaves in a saucepan and cook over medium heat until the vegetables are tender, about 15 minutes. Remove the bay leaves. Add the remaining ingredients. Blend the soup in batches in a blender or food processor until smooth. Serve at once, or reheat just before serving.

Cream of Celery Soup

SERVINGS: 8
PREPARATION TIME: 30 MINUTES
COOKING TIME: 45 MINUTES

A rich, creamy soup because of the cashew pieces. To make a lighter version, substitute low-fat soy or rice milk for the cashews.

5 stalks celery with tops, chopped
1 large onion, chopped
2 medium carrots, scrubbed and grated
2 medium potatoes, peeled and cubed
9 cups water
⅔ cup raw cashew pieces
⅓ cup whole-wheat pastry flour
⅓ cup soy sauce
¼ cup chopped fresh parsley
Pinch dried dill
Pinch cayenne
Freshly ground black pepper to taste

Place the celery, onion, carrots, and potatoes in a large soup pot with 8 cups of the water and simmer until tender, about 30 minutes. Place the remaining 1 cup water, the cashew pieces, and the whole-wheat pastry flour in a blender and puree. (You can substitute 2 cups of low-fat soy milk or rice milk for the 1 cup of water and cashews.) Add 4 cups of the cooked vegetables to the blender mixture and puree. Pour this mixture into the pot and bring to a boil, stirring until the soup thickens. Add the soy sauce, parsley, dill, cayenne, and black pepper. Cook for 5 minutes to blend the flavors.

Sweet Squash Soup

SERVINGS: 8 TO 10
PREPARATION TIME: 30 MINUTES
COOKING TIME: 45 MINUTES

This soup freezes well. It's a delicious autumn supper served with Curried Rice Salad or Fruited Wild Rice Salad and a loaf of fresh whole-wheat bread.

1 large butternut or buttercup squash
1½ cups sliced onion
1½ cups peeled and chopped apple

1 cup chopped carrot
2 to 3 teaspoons minced fresh ginger
5 cups water

Put the whole squash in a microwave oven and cook on high power for 8 minutes. Peel the squash and cut into cubes. (If you don't have a microwave oven, this step may be omitted. This brief cooking time simply makes the squash easier to peel and cut up.)

Place all of the ingredients in a large soup pot and simmer over medium-low heat for 45 minutes. Place the soup in a blender or food processor, in batches, and blend until smooth and creamy.

Spicy Carrot Soup

SERVINGS: 6
PREPARATION TIME: 20 MINUTES
COOKING TIME: 30 MINUTES

2 quarts vegetable broth
6 medium carrots, scrubbed and thinly sliced
2 large onions, chopped
2 medium red potatoes, peeled and chopped
1 cup chopped celery

1 teaspoon ground cumin
1 teaspoon curry powder
2 tablespoons fresh lemon juice
Chopped fresh watercress for garnish

In a large soup pot, combine all of the ingredients except the lemon juice and watercress. Bring to a boil, cover, and reduce the heat. Simmer until the vegetables are tender, about 30 minutes. Add the lemon juice. Puree the soup, a portion at a time, in a blender or food processor. Place in a soup tureen and garnish with watercress.

Onion Soup Provençale

SERVINGS: 8

PREPARATION TIME: 15 MINUTES

COOKING TIME: 1 HOUR

This soup is excellent served with Easy Nonfat Garlic Bread.

5 cups water

4 large onions, sliced and separated into rings

2 small zucchini, sliced

1 medium eggplant, peeled and chopped, or 2 small Japanese eggplants, sliced

1 to 2 cl garlic, crushed

One 6- omato pa

½ cup e (optional)

¼ cup pped fresh basil

2 tablespoons soy sauce

Freshly ground pepper to taste

Combine all of the ingredients in a large soup pot. Bring to a boil, cover, reduce the heat, and simmer over medium-low heat for about 1 hour, or until the vegetables are tender.

Garlic Soup

SERVINGS: 10 TO 12
PREPARATION TIME: 30 MINUTES
COOKING TIME: 1 TO 1¼ HOURS

3 quarts water
25 to 30 whole cloves garlic, papery coverings removed
½ cup barley
¼ cup wild rice
4 onions, chopped
4 potatoes, peeled and chunked
4 carrots, scrubbed and sliced
3 stalks celery, sliced
4 tablespoons soy sauce
1 teaspoon dried thyme
1 teaspoon freshly ground pepper

Place 2 cups of the water in a large soup pot. Add the whole garlic cloves and cook over medium heat for 15 minutes. Remove the garlic cloves and mash them thoroughly before proceeding. (Use a potato masher or process in a blender or food processor.)

Add the remaining 2½ quarts water, the barley, and the wild rice. Bring to a boil, cover, and cook for 15 minutes. Add the remaining ingredients and continue to cook until tender, 30 to 45 minutes.

This soup tastes best if allowed to cool and then reheated. Make it several days ahead, or make with the intention of freezing for later use.

Green Gnocchi Soup

SERVINGS: 4 TO 6
PREPARATION TIME: 15 MINUTES
COOKING TIME: 25 MINUTES

1½ quarts water
1 small onion, chopped
¼ cup chopped scallion
6 cups finely chopped
   greens (spinach, escarole,
   mustard greens,
   watercress, etc.)

1 medium chayote, peeled
   and chopped (see
   Note)
½ pound gnocchi (Ferrara
   brand is a good one)
Freshly ground pepper for
   garnish

Place ½ cup of the water in a large soup pot. Add the onion and scallion and sauté until the onion is soft, about 4 minutes. Add the greens, cover, and cook over low heat until they are soft, about 4 minutes. Add the remaining 5½ cups water and the chayote. Bring to a boil, cover, and simmer until the chayote is tender, about 15 minutes.

Puree the soup a portion at a time in a blender or food processor. Return to the pan and keep warm. Meanwhile, cook the gnocchi according to the package directions. Add to the pureed soup. Serve at once, garnished with freshly ground pepper.

Note: Chayote squash is a light green, pear-shaped, mild-tasting squash. It can usually be found in most supermarkets in summer and fall. Zucchini could be substituted if chayote is unavailable, but the flavor of the soup will be less distinct.

Spinach-Mushroom Soup

SERVINGS: 4 TO 6
PREPARATION TIME: 15 MINUTES
COOKING TIME: 20 MINUTES

1 large onion, thinly
    sliced
1½ pounds mushrooms,
    thinly sliced
¼ cup white wine
1 quart water or vegetable
    broth
One 3.5-ounce package enoki
    mushrooms (see Note)

2 tablespoons soy sauce
4 cups packed washed
    spinach leaves, cut into
    thin strips
Freshly ground pepper
    to taste

Place the onion and mushrooms in a large saucepan with the wine.
Cook slowly over low heat for about 10 minutes. Add the water or
vegetable broth, the enoki mushrooms, and the soy sauce. Cook for
an additional 10 minutes. Stir in the spinach and season with the
pepper. Turn off the heat. Serve as soon as the spinach is wilted.

Note: Enoki mushrooms are very small, white mushrooms with a
longish thin stem (2 to 3 inches). They are very delicate and mild
in flavor, and are sold in some supermarkets and Asian markets. If
you are unable to find them, just omit them from the recipe.

Sopa Seca (Dry Soup)

SERVINGS: 4
PREPARATION TIME: 15 MINUTES
COOKING TIME: 15 MINUTES

This soup is Mexican in origin. It really does not look like a soup at all because all the liquid is absorbed. Serve this as a first course with burritos or enchiladas.

8 ounces coiled vermicelli
¼ cup water
1 small onion, chopped
1 clove garlic, crushed
One 4-ounce can diced green chilies
2½ cups vegetable broth

2 medium tomatoes, chopped
Freshly ground black pepper for garnish
Chopped fresh cilantro for garnish

Place the vermicelli in a plastic bag. Take a rolling pin and roll over the bag until the noodles are crumbled. Set aside.

Place the water in a large skillet or wok. Add the onion, garlic, and chilies. Cook, stirring, until softened, about 2 minutes. Add the vermicelli and vegetable broth. Bring to a boil, reduce the heat, cover, and cook for 5 minutes. Add the tomato, stir, and continue to cook, uncovered, over low heat until all of the liquid is absorbed. Garnish with freshly ground black pepper and chopped cilantro.

Variation: Add ½ cup corn kernels and ½ cup thawed frozen or fresh green peas to the mixture along with the noodles and broth.

Twin Sisters Vegetable Soup

SERVINGS: 8
PREPARATION TIME: 40 MINUTES (NEED COOKED BEANS)
COOKING TIME: 70 MINUTES

This recipe came from a friend who got the recipe from a restaurant called Twin Sisters. She liked it so much she asked them to share it with me. This soup tastes best when made a day ahead and reheated.

1 medium onion, chopped
2 cloves garlic, chopped fine or pressed
2 teaspoons dried oregano
⅛ teaspoon freshly ground pepper
2 Idaho potatoes, scrubbed and unpeeled
1 zucchini

1 large yellow squash
3 stalks celery
2 carrots, scrubbed and unpeeled
3 tomatoes
2 bay leaves
1 cup cooked kidney or pinto beans

Sauté the onion, garlic, oregano, and pepper in a small amount of water until the onion is translucent, about 5 minutes. Set aside.

Dice the remaining vegetables, except the tomatoes, and place them in a large pot; add the sautéed onion mixture. Add water just to cover the vegetables. Add the bay leaves, bring to a boil, and reduce the heat. Simmer until the vegetables are just tender, 10 to 15 minutes.

Place the tomatoes in a blender or food processor and process until pureed. Pour into a saucepan and gently boil for 20 minutes to remove any acidic taste. Add the tomatoes to the soup, along with the cooked beans.

Cook for 30 minutes over low heat. Refrigerate overnight to allow the flavors to "marry." Reheat and serve the next day.

Variation: One-half cup each of corn and green beans can also be added to the soup.

Tomato-Onion Soup with Rigatoni

SERVINGS: 4
PREPARATION TIME: 10 MINUTES
COOKING TIME: 1¼ HOURS

1 large onion, chopped
⅛ teaspoon garlic powder
1 cup water
One 28-ounce can whole
    tomatoes, chopped, with
    their liquid

1 tablespoon dried parsley
1 cup rigatoni
½ teaspoon dried thyme
1 bay leaf
½ teaspoon dried basil
1 tablespoon soy sauce

Sauté the onion and garlic powder in the water for 15 minutes. Add the remaining ingredients, except the soy sauce. Simmer, covered, for 1 hour. Add the soy sauce and remove the bay leaf just before serving.

Green Bean Soup

SERVINGS: 6 TO 8
PREPARATION TIME: 35 MINUTES
COOKING TIME: 30 MINUTES

This is a surprising soup, wonderful for a first course. It is very light and refreshing, full of the flavor of fresh green beans. Make it when green beans are in season or you have a garden full of them. Do not make this with frozen or canned beans.

1 large onion, chopped
6 cups fresh green beans, chopped into 1½-inch pieces
6 cups water
2 tablespoons soy sauce

1 teaspoon dried basil
½ teaspoon dried marjoram
¼ teaspoon celery seed
Several twists freshly ground pepper

Place the onion and beans in a large pot with the water. Bring to a boil, reduce the heat, and add the remaining ingredients. Cover and cook over medium heat for 30 minutes. Remove from the heat and puree the soup in batches in a blender or food processor. Serve immediately.

Vegetable Soup

SERVINGS: 8
PREPARATION TIME: 30 MINUTES (NEED COOKED BEANS)
COOKING TIME: 45 MINUTES

¼ cup water
1 large onion, chopped
1 clove garlic, crushed
1 cup chopped celery
One 28-ounce can whole
  tomatoes, chopped, with
  their liquid
2 quarts water
1 cup chopped carrot
2 cups chopped zucchini
2 cups shredded cabbage
3 cups cooked beans
  (kidney, garbanzo,
  white, black, etc.)

1 tablespoon dried parsley
1 teaspoon dried basil
1 teaspoon dried sage
1 teaspoon dried chervil
  Dash ground cinnamon
1 cup frozen green peas
1 cup frozen chopped
  green beans
1 package frozen chopped
  spinach
1 cup whole-wheat pasta
½ tablespoon fresh lemon
  juice
⅛ cup raisins

Place the ¼ cup water in a large soup pot. Add the onion, garlic, and celery. Cook, stirring, over medium heat for 5 minutes. Add the tomatoes and 2 quarts of water. Bring to a boil. Add the carrot, zucchini, cabbage, cooked beans, and spices. Cover and simmer for 20 minutes. Add the frozen vegetables and pasta. Bring to a boil and simmer, uncovered, for about 15 minutes. Stir in the lemon juice and raisins. Serve.

Vegetable-Market Soup with Millet and Shredded Greens

SERVINGS: 8 TO 10

PREPARATION TIME: 45 MINUTES   COOKING TIME: 55 MINUTES

1½ cups water
¼ cup millet
3 medium onions, chopped
3 leeks, washed and sliced
1 medium turnip, peeled and chopped
2 cups chopped carrot
2 cups chopped zucchini
2 cups peeled and chopped red potato
1½ cups chopped celery
4 large cloves garlic, sliced
8 cups vegetable broth (page 132) or water
2 large tomatoes, chopped

1 small jalapeño pepper, seeded and minced (optional)
2 tablespoons soy sauce
½ teaspoon chopped fresh thyme
½ teaspoon chopped fresh marjoram
1 cup low-fat soy milk
¼ teaspoon ground nutmeg
Freshly ground black pepper
2 cups shredded greens (bok choy, escarole, arugula, or spinach)

Place 1 cup of the water in a small saucepan with the millet. Bring to a boil, reduce the heat, cover, and simmer for 20 to 25 minutes, until the millet is tender and the liquid is absorbed. Remove from the heat and set aside.

Meanwhile, place the remaining ½ cup of water in a large soup pot. Add the onions and cook, stirring, for several minutes, until softened. Add next thirteen ingredients (up to but not including the soy milk). Bring to a boil, reduce the heat, cover partially, and simmer for about 45 minutes.

Remove the soup from the pan and puree in batches in a blender or food processor. Return to the pan. Stir in the soy milk, nutmeg, and pepper to taste. Add the cooked millet and the greens. Cover and simmer until the greens wilt, about 4 minutes. Serve at once.

Note: This soup freezes well, so even though it makes a lot, you'll have another meal for later.

Vegetable Chowder

SERVINGS: 6 TO 8
PREPARATION TIME: 30 MINUTES
COOKING TIME: 45 MINUTES

3½ cups water
1 medium onion, chopped
2 cloves garlic, minced
2 stalks celery, sliced
2 carrots, scrubbed and chopped
1 medium green bell pepper, chopped
2 large potatoes, peeled and chopped

3 tablespoons soy sauce
1 tablespoon thinly sliced fresh basil
¼ to ½ teaspoon white pepper
2 cups frozen corn kernels
2 medium tomatoes, seeded and chopped
3 cups low-fat soy milk

Place ½ cup of the water in a large pot. Add the onion, garlic, celery, carrots, and green pepper. Cook, stirring, over medium-low heat for 5 minutes. Add the remaining 3 cups of water, the soy sauce, basil, and pepper. Cover and cook for 20 minutes.

Add the corn and cook for an additional 10 minutes. Add the tomatoes and soy milk. Cook 10 minutes longer and serve at once.

Variation: Before adding the tomatoes and soy milk, puree half of the soup in a blender or food processor. Return to the pan and proceed as directed.

Leslie's Vegetable-Bean Soup

SERVINGS: 10 TO 12
PREPARATION TIME: 40 MINUTES
COOKING TIME: 1½ HOURS

The woman who sent us this recipe named it after her husband because it is his favorite soup.

3½ quarts water
12 ounces tomato paste
2 tablespoons oil-free Italian dressing
1 large red onion, finely minced
2 bunches scallions, chopped
4 cloves garlic, minced
5 stalks celery, chopped
¾ cup chopped fresh parsley
½ head cabbage, chopped
1 green bell pepper, chopped

4 large carrots, scrubbed and chopped
4 medium zucchini, chopped
½ pound mushrooms, sliced
4 peeled tomatoes, chopped (or one 15-ounce can chopped tomatoes)
One 15-ounce can each of kidney beans, corn, and green beans, rinsed and drained
2 cups whole-wheat macaroni

Place the water, tomato paste, and dressing in a large pot. Add the chopped vegetables and simmer over low heat for about 1 hour. Add the canned beans and vegetables and the macaroni. Continue to cook until the macaroni is tender, 20 to 30 minutes.

Note: This makes a large amount of soup. Freeze half for use on another day.

Mixed Bean and Vegetable Soup

SERVINGS: 8 TO 10
PREPARATION TIME: 40 MINUTES
COOKING TIME: 3 HOURS

2 cups assorted dried
   beans (kidney, pinto,
   black, Great Northern,
   black-eyed peas,
   lentils, split peas; see
   Note)
2 quarts water
1 onion, thinly sliced
1 leek, washed and
   thinly sliced
2 potatoes, peeled and
   thinly sliced
1 carrot, scrubbed and
   thinly sliced
3 stalks celery, thinly
   sliced

1 zucchini, thinly sliced
¼ pound mushrooms,
   sliced
2 cloves garlic, minced
2 tomatoes, seeded and
   chopped
2 bay leaves
2 teaspoons dried basil
1½ teaspoon dried
   oregano
½ teaspoon dried
   marjoram
¼ to ½ teaspoon freshly
   ground pepper
¼ teaspoon dried savory

Place the beans and water in a large soup pot. Bring to a boil,
cover, and cook over medium heat until the beans are almost tender, about 2 hours. Add the remaining ingredients and continue to
cook until the vegetables are tender, 40 to 60 minutes. Remove the
bay leaves before serving.

Note: If you soak the beans overnight, the total cooking time may
be reduced by 30 minutes.

Mediterranean White Bean Soup

SERVINGS: 6 TO 8

PREPARATION TIME: 15 MINUTES   COOKING TIME: 2½ TO 3 HOURS

2 cups white beans (see Note)
7 cups water
1 onion, chopped
6 to 7 cloves garlic, minced
2 potatoes, peeled and chopped
One 8-ounce can water-packed artichokes, drained
One 4-ounce can sliced black olives, drained
One 8-ounce can tomato sauce
1 teaspoon Italian herb mix

Place the beans in a large pot with the water. Cover and cook over medium heat for 1 hour. Add the onion and garlic and continue to cook until the beans are tender, 1 to 1½ hours. Add the potatoes and cook for another 20 minutes. Add the remaining ingredients and cook for about 10 more minutes.

Note: If you soak the beans overnight, the total cooking time may be reduced by 30 minutes.

White Bean Minestrone

SERVINGS: 8

PREPARATION TIME: 20 MINUTES (PLUS 1 HOUR STANDING TIME)
COOKING TIME: 2 HOURS, 45 MINUTES

1 cup white beans
2 quarts water
2 cups chopped celery
One 15-ounce can whole tomatoes, chopped, with their liquid
1 cup peeled and chopped yellow turnip
¼ cup chopped fresh parsley
1 teaspoon dried basil
4 cups shredded cabbage
2 large zucchini, sliced
½ cup whole-wheat elbows

Place the beans and 1 quart of the water in a saucepan. Heat to boiling, cook for 2 minutes, and remove from the heat. Cover and let stand for 1 hour.

Place the celery in a large soup pot. Add about ½ cup of the remaining water and sauté until the celery softens. Add the tomatoes, turnip, parsley, basil, the remaining 3½ cups water, and the beans and their liquid. Cover. Heat slowly to boiling and simmer for 2 hours.

Add the cabbage and zucchini. Simmer for 30 minutes. Add the elbows and simmer for another 15 minutes.

Creamy White Bean Soup

SERVINGS: 6 TO 8
PREPARATION TIME: 15 MINUTES, PLUS 1 HOUR STANDING TIME
COOKING TIME: 3 HOURS

1 pound white beans (Great Northern work the best)
2 quarts water
1 onion, chopped
1 leek, white part only, washed and sliced
3 cloves garlic, pressed
1 potato, peeled and chopped
1 bay leaf
½ teaspoon dried sage
Freshly ground pepper
Chopped fresh parsley (optional)

Place the beans and water in a large soup pot. Bring to a boil, turn off the heat, and let rest for 1 hour. Add the onion, leek, and garlic. Bring to a boil again, cover, and cook over medium heat for 1 hour. Add the potato and seasonings. Cook for an additional 2 hours, or until the beans are tender. Remove the bay leaf.

Puree the soup in batches in a blender or food processor. Return to the pot and thin out slightly with ½ to 1 cup of hot water. Add freshly ground pepper to taste. Garnish with chopped fresh parsley, if desired.

Texas-Style Black-Eyed Pea Soup

SERVINGS: 6
PREPARATION TIME: 20 MINUTES
COOKING TIME: 1 HOUR, 25 MINUTES

The woman who sent me this recipe says she has been making this soup for years. It is delicious and adapts to different tastes. Add some cooked rice or pasta for a change, or vary the seasonings to suit your family.

One 20-ounce package frozen black-eyed peas
4¾ cups water
1 large onion, chopped
One 28-ounce can crushed tomatoes
1 teaspoon ground ginger
3 to 4 carrots, scrubbed and sliced
4 to 5 stalks celery, diced
1 medium potato, peeled and diced
1 clove garlic, minced

Place the black-eyed peas in a nonstick frying pan with ½ cup of the water. Sauté the peas until thawed, stirring occasionally, about 5 minutes. Transfer the peas and water to a large soup pot. Add the onion, tomatoes, ginger, and 4 cups of the water. Cook over medium-low heat for 45 minutes, stirring occasionally.

Place the remaining ¼ cup water in the nonstick frying pan. Add the carrots, celery, potato, and garlic. Cook, stirring for 5 minutes. Add to the peas, onions and tomatoes, cover, and simmer for another 30 minutes.

Grandma Gibson's Split Pea Soup

SERVINGS: 8 TO 10
PREPARATION TIME: 25 MINUTES
COOKING TIME: 1½ HOURS

The woman who sent us this recipe said that she took her grandmother's recipe for pea soup, modified it slightly, and liked the result even more than the original.

2 cups green split peas
2 quarts water
1 large onion, chopped
2 large carrots, scrubbed and chopped
6 stalks celery, chopped
5 to 6 cloves garlic, minced
1 bay leaf
¼ teaspoon dried thyme
Freshly ground pepper to taste

4 large potatoes, peeled and chopped
One 15-ounce can tomato sauce
1 to 2 tablespoons chili sauce, or to taste (see Note 1)
Chopped fresh parsley for garnish

Place the peas and water in a large soup pot. Bring to a boil, reduce the heat, cover, and simmer for 30 minutes. Add the onion, carrot, celery, garlic, bay leaf, and thyme. Simmer for another 30 minutes. Add the remaining ingredients, except the parsley, and cook for an additional 30 minutes. Remove the bay leaf and garnish with parsley before serving.

Notes: 1. Chili sauce is found in the Oriental section of most supermarkets. It is also called ground chili paste. Use it sparingly—it is very hot.

2. This soup freezes well.

Lentil-Tomato Soup

SERVINGS: 10
PREPARATION TIME: 20 MINUTES
COOKING TIME: 2 HOURS

1½ cups lentils
8 cups water or vegetable broth
1 bay leaf
½ teaspoon dried thyme
¼ teaspoon dried sage
1 large red onion, diced
2 stalks celery, sliced

2 cloves garlic, minced
One 15-ounce can whole tomatoes, chopped, with liquid
2 tablespoons minced fresh mint
Freshly ground pepper to taste

Place the lentils in a large soup pot. Add the water or vegetable stock. Bring to a boil. Add the bay leaf, thyme, and sage. Reduce the heat to low, cover, and cook for 1 hour.

Add the onion, celery, garlic, and tomatoes. Continue to cook for another 45 minutes. Add the mint and the pepper. Cook for an additional 15 minutes.

Curried Red Lentil Soup

SERVINGS: 8
PREPARATION TIME: 10 MINUTES
COOKING TIME: 1 HOUR, 10 MINUTES

2 cups chopped onion
2 cloves garlic, minced
7½ cups water
1 teaspoon ground turmeric
¾ teaspoon ground cumin
½ teaspoon ground ginger
¼ teaspoon freshly ground black pepper

⅛ teaspoon cayenne
1½ cups red lentils
1 teaspoon red-wine vinegar
2 tablespoons chopped fresh parsley

Sauté the onion and garlic in ½ cup of the water in a large pot until the onion is soft, about 5 minutes. Add the seasonings and cook for 1 minute. Add the lentils and the remaining water. Bring to a boil, reduce the heat, cover, and simmer for 1 hour. Stir in the vinegar. Garnish with parsley before serving.

Adas Bi Sabaanikh
(Lentil and Spinach Soup)

SERVINGS: 6
PREPARATION TIME: 30 MINUTES
COOKING TIME: 1 HOUR, 10 MINUTES

This is a Middle Eastern soup, typical of the simple foods served in the desert regions. Serve with pita bread and a grain or vegetable dish for a simple meal. This soup is also good served cold, stuffed into pita bread.

1½ cups lentils	½ cup chopped fresh parsley
8 cups water	
1 large onion, chopped	¼ teaspoon freshly ground black pepper
2 to 3 cloves garlic, crushed	
2 bunches spinach, cleaned and chopped	⅛ teaspoon crushed red pepper flakes
	¼ cup fresh lemon juice

Place the lentils and water in a large pot. Bring to a boil, cover, and cook for 30 minutes over medium-low heat. Add the onion and garlic and cook for an additional 30 minutes. Add the spinach, parsley, and peppers. Mix well and cook for another 10 minutes. Add the lemon juice just before serving. Mix in well and serve at once.

Split Pea and Lentil Soup
with Vegetables

SERVINGS: 8

PREPARATION TIME: 15 MINUTES   COOKING TIME: 55 MINUTES

1½ cups chopped onion
1 cup chopped celery
2 cloves garlic, minced
8 cups water
1 cup diced carrot
1 bay leaf
1 tablespoon soy sauce

¼ teaspoon freshly ground
    black pepper
¼ teaspoon dried rosemary,
    crushed
½ pound (1⅛ cups) green
    split peas
½ pound (1⅛ cups) lentils

In a large saucepan, sauté the onion, celery, and garlic in ½ cup of the water until the vegetables are tender, about 5 minutes. Add the carrot, the remaining 7½ cups water, bay leaf, soy sauce, pepper, and rosemary. Heat to boiling. Stir in the peas and lentils. Simmer, covered, for 45 minutes, stirring occasionally.

Drunken Bean Soup

SERVINGS: 6

PREPARATION TIME: 15 MINUTES   COOKING TIME: 30 MINUTES

This is actually a thick bean stew. It tastes best if it's made early in the day or the day before, then reheated. Serve with corn or flour tortillas.

Two 15-ounce cans pinto
    beans, drained and
    rinsed
½ cup water or beer
½ medium onion, sliced

2 to 3 cloves garlic, minced
½ cup fresh cilantro
    leaves
1 fresh jalapeño pepper,
    thinly sliced

Combine all of the ingredients in a saucepan. Simmer over low heat for 30 minutes.

Southwestern Black Bean Soup

SERVINGS: 8 TO 10

PREPARATION TIME: 15 MINUTES, PLUS OVERNIGHT SOAKING OF BEANS
COOKING TIME: 3 HOURS

1 pound black beans
2 quarts water
1 large onion, coarsely chopped
1 to 2 cloves garlic, minced
Two 16-ounce cans whole tomatoes, chopped, with liquid
One 4-ounce can chopped green chilies

1 teaspoon ground cumin
1 teaspoon chili powder
1 teaspoon fresh lemon juice
¼ teaspoon crushed red pepper flakes
¼ cup chopped fresh cilantro

Soak the beans overnight in the water.

Bring to a boil in the soaking water, cover, and reduce the heat. Simmer for 1 hour, then add the remaining ingredients, except the cilantro. Cook until the beans are tender, about 2 hours. Add the cilantro just before serving. Mix it in well and let the soup rest, covered, for about 15 minutes. Serve hot.

Note: This is great to make in a slow cooker. Put everything into the pot, except the cilantro, early in the morning. (No need to soak the beans first.) Set the cooker on high, cover, and let it cook all day. Add the cilantro just before serving.

Black Bean Soup with Cilantro and Orange

SERVINGS: 6 TO 8

PREPARATION TIME: 30 MINUTES, PLUS OVERNIGHT SOAKING OF BEANS

COOKING TIME: 2 TO 3 HOURS

2 cups black beans
8 cups water
2 tablespoons vegetable broth/seasoning mix
Freshly ground pepper to taste
2 leeks, washed and sliced

2 carrots, scrubbed and chopped
1 onion, chopped
¼ to ½ cup chopped fresh cilantro
Grated zest of 1 orange

Soak the beans overnight in enough water to cover. Drain. Place the beans, 6 cups of water, broth mix, and pepper in a large pot and cook over low heat until the beans are tender, about 2 to 3 hours. Meanwhile, cook the leek, carrot, and onion in about 2 cups of water until tender, about 30 minutes.

When the beans are done, remove 2 cups of beans in liquid and process in a blender or food processor until smooth. Return to the soup pot. Place the cooked vegetables and water in the blender or processor and process until smooth. Add to the beans and mix well. Stir in the cilantro and orange zest just before serving.

Variations: Cook 1 peeled and chopped potato with the beans and/or puree all of the bean mixture for a thicker soup.

Spicy Garbanzo Bean Soup

SERVINGS: 8 TO 10
PREPARATION TIME: 15 MINUTES, PLUS 1 HOUR STANDING TIME
COOKING TIME: 4 HOURS

1 cup garbanzo beans
3 quarts water
1 onion, coarsely chopped
2 potatoes, scrubbed and diced
One 28-ounce can whole tomatoes, chopped, with liquid
½ cup chopped fresh parsley
1 teaspoon ground turmeric

1 teaspoon ground cumin
¼ to ½ teaspoon freshly ground black pepper
½ teaspoon ground ginger
⅛ teaspoon powdered saffron
Dash cayenne
¼ cup fresh lemon juice (optional)
¼ cup chopped fresh cilantro

Place the beans and water in a large soup pot. Bring to a boil, turn off the heat, and let rest for 1 hour. Add the onion, bring to a boil again, cover, and cook over medium heat for 3 hours. Add the remaining ingredients except for the lemon juice and cilantro. Cook for 1 more hour. Stir in the lemon juice and cilantro just before serving.

Note: This soup freezes well.

Lima Bean Soup

SERVINGS: 8
PREPARATION TIME: 15 MINUTES
COOKING TIME: 4 HOURS

Serve with cornbread.

1½ cups dry lima beans
8 cups water
2 onions, chopped
3 cloves garlic, chopped
2 teaspoons of your favorite dried herbs (e.g., basil, oregano, and parsley; cumin and curry; marjoram, thyme, and parsley; Italian herb blend (Parsley Patch); Mexican blend (Parsley Patch)

2 large potatoes, peeled and chopped
2 cups frozen lima beans

Combine the dry lima beans, water, onion, garlic, and herbs in a large saucepan and simmer until the beans are almost tender, about 3 to 3½ hours. Add the potatoes and the frozen lima beans and simmer for ½ hour, or until the vegetables and beans are tender.

Note: The cooking time can be shortened by 30 minutes by pre-soaking the dry lima beans overnight.

Spicy Mixed Bean Soup

SERVINGS: 8

PREPARATION TIME: 15 MINUTES, PLUS 1 HOUR STANDING TIME

COOKING TIME: 3 TO 4 HOURS

¼ cup of each of the following: black beans; kidney beans; white beans; garbanzo beans; lentils; split green peas; baby lima beans; and barley

2 quarts water

1 large onion, chopped

2 cloves garlic, crushed

One 16-ounce can tomato sauce

One 16-ounce can whole tomatoes, chopped, with liquid

¼ cup chopped canned mild green chilies

1 teaspoon chili powder

¼ teaspoon crushed red pepper flakes

Place all of the beans in a large soup pot with the water. Bring to a boil. Boil for 2 minutes, remove from the heat, and let rest for 1 hour. (Or soak the beans overnight in water to cover and eliminate the previous step.) Add the remaining ingredients. Bring to a boil (in the soaking water if so prepared), cover, reduce the heat, and cook until the beans are tender, 3 to 4 hours.

Note: This soup is wonderful to make in a slow cooker. Add all of the ingredients at once. Cook on high for 8 to 10 hours or on low for 20 hours.

Stews

Okra Gumbo

SERVINGS: 6 TO 8
PREPARATION TIME: 15 MINUTES
COOKING TIME: 1 HOUR

Serve in a bowl by itself or over brown rice or other whole grains.

1 cup chopped onion
1 cup chopped green bell pepper
1 cup chopped celery
2 cups water
3 cloves garlic, minced
One 15-ounce can whole tomatoes, chopped, with liquid
One 8-ounce can tomato sauce
One 4-ounce can chopped green chilies

2 tablespoons chopped fresh parsley
1 bay leaf
¼ teaspoon dried thyme
¼ teaspoon paprika
¼ teaspoon freshly ground pepper
⅛ teaspoon cayenne
1½ cups sliced fresh okra
2 tablespoons cornstarch, mixed with ¼ cup cold water

Place the onion, green pepper, and celery in a large pot with ½ cup of the water. Sauté over medium heat, stirring occasionally, until the vegetables are tender, about 10 minutes. Add the remaining 1½ cups water, along with the garlic, tomatoes, tomato sauce, chilies, parsley, and spices. Cover, reduce the heat, and simmer over low heat for 30 minutes.

Stir in the okra and cook for an additional 15 to 20 minutes, or until the okra is tender. Gradually add the cornstarch mixture while stirring. Cook, stirring, until thickened slightly.

Hearty Brown Stew

SERVINGS: 6 TO 8
PREPARATION TIME: 25 MINUTES
COOKING TIME: 1 HOUR

2 onions, sliced
2 stalks celery, thickly
    sliced
2 carrots, scrubbed and
    thickly sliced
3 potatoes, scrubbed and
    chunked
1 green bell pepper, cut
    into strips
½ pound mushrooms,
    quartered
2 to 3 cloves garlic
2 cups water

¼ cup low-sodium soy
    sauce
¼ cup tomato juice
½ tablespoon grated fresh
    ginger
½ teaspoon dried
    marjoram
½ teaspoon dried thyme
½ teaspoon paprika
3 to 4 tablespoons cornstarch
    or arrowroot, mixed
    with ½ cup cold water

Combine all of the ingredients, except the cornstarch or arrowroot mixture, in a large pot. Bring to a boil, lower the heat, cover, and simmer for about 1 hour, or until the vegetables are tender. Add the cornstarch or arrowroot mixture to the stew. Stir until thickened.

Note: This can also be made in a slow cooker. Follow the above directions. Cook on high for 6 hours or on low for 12 hours. Add the cornstarch or arrowroot mixture just before serving and stir until thickened.

Cajun Black-Eyed Pea Stew

SERVINGS: 2

PREPARATION TIME: 15 MINUTES (PLUS OVERNIGHT SOAKING)

COOKING TIME: 1 HOUR

Serve over brown rice or another whole grain.

½ cup black-eyed peas
1 onion, sliced
One 14-ounce can Cajun-
style stewed tomatoes
2 cloves garlic, chopped
2 tablespoons soy sauce

3 tablespoons catsup
2 teaspoons Cajun Spices
(page 345)
⅛ teaspoon Tabasco
¾ cup water

Soak the black-eyed peas overnight in water to cover. Drain. Place all of the ingredients in a medium saucepan. Cook until the peas are tender, about 1 hour.

Ratatouille

SERVINGS: 8

PREPARATION TIME: 20 MINUTES   COOKING TIME: 45 TO 60 MINUTES

Serve this stuffed into pita bread, on its own as a stew, or over potatoes or whole grains.

½ cup water
2 large onions, chopped
2 to 4 cloves garlic, minced
2 large eggplants, cut into
1-inch chunks
6 zucchini, thickly sliced
2 bell peppers (green or
red), cut into 1-inch
chunks
4 cups chopped fresh
tomatoes

15 fresh basil leaves,
chopped
3 tablespoons chopped
fresh parsley
1 tablespoon chopped
fresh thyme
Freshly ground black
pepper to taste

Place the water, onions, and garlic in a large pot. Cook, stirring, over medium heat until the onion softens slightly. Add the eggplants; cook, stirring, for 5 minutes. Add the zucchini and peppers and cook for an additional 5 minutes. Add the tomato; stir well. Cover and cook over medium-low heat for 30 to 45 minutes, depending on whether you like your vegetables crunchy or softened. Add the fresh seasonings about 5 minutes before the end of the cooking time. Stir to mix in well. Serve hot or cold.

Squash and Tomato Stew

SERVINGS: 8
PREPARATION TIME: 25 MINUTES
COOKING TIME: 45 MINUTES

1 tablespoon soy sauce
1 cup water
2 large onions, finely chopped
2 cloves garlic, minced
1 pound tomatoes, peeled, seeded, and chopped (see Note)
1 tablespoon chopped fresh oregano

¼ teaspoon freshly ground pepper
4 pounds butternut squash, peeled, seeded, and cut into 1-inch cubes
2 cups frozen corn kernels
1 cup frozen green peas
Chopped fresh parsley for garnish

Place the soy sauce and ½ cup of the water in a large soup pot. Heat to boiling. Add the onions and garlic. Cook, stirring, until softened slightly. Add the tomatoes, oregano, and pepper. Cook until the tomatoes are tender, stirring occasionally, about 3 minutes. Add the remaining ½ cup water and the squash. Cover and simmer until the squash is tender, about 30 minutes.

Add the corn and peas. Cook for another 2 minutes. Garnish with parsley before serving.

Note: To peel tomatoes, dip briefly in boiling water until the skins loosen, then slip the skins off.

Spicy Yam Stew

SERVINGS: 8 TO 10
PREPARATION TIME: 25 MINUTES
COOKING TIME: 35 MINUTES

Serve over whole grains or pasta, or in a bowl by itself.

1½ cups vegetable broth (page 132) or water
2 medium sweet potatoes or yams, peeled and cubed
2 cups celery, sliced on the diagonal
1 green bell pepper, coarsely chopped
1 large onion, coarsely chopped
2 medium carrots, scrubbed, quartered and chopped into 1-inch chunks
One 16-ounce can whole tomatoes, chopped
One 3-inch piece stick cinnamon
1 to 2 tablespoons low-sodium soy sauce
Freshly ground black pepper to taste
Pinch cayenne
2 tablespoons arrowroot (or cornstarch), dissolved in 2 tablespoons cold water
¼ cup chopped fresh parsley for garnish

Place all of the ingredients, except the arrowroot or cornstarch mixture and the parsley, in a large soup pot and cook, covered, over medium-low heat for 30 minutes or until all of the vegetables are tender, stirring occasionally. Add the arrowroot or cornstarch mixture, stir until thickened, and adjust the seasonings to taste. Garnish with parsley.

Note: This can also be made in a slow cooker. Follow the above directions. Cook for 6 to 8 hours on low power. Add the arrowroot or cornstarch before serving.

Spicy Vegetable Stew

SERVINGS: 6
PREPARATION TIME: 20 MINUTES
COOKING TIME: 1 HOUR

Serve this stew as is or over rice or mashed potatoes.

3 potatoes, peeled and chopped
1 zucchini, sliced
1 onion, sliced
1 cup frozen corn kernels
1 cup broccoflower (or cauliflower) florets
1 green bell pepper, chopped into large pieces
2 carrots, scrubbed and sliced
Two 4-ounce cans chopped green chilies
One 16-ounce can whole tomatoes, chopped, with liquid
1 tablespoon diced jalapeño pepper
2 cups water

Mix all of the ingredients together in a large soup pot and simmer over low heat until the vegetables are tender, about 1 hour.

Note: This recipe can also be made in a slow cooker. Cook on low power for 8 to 10 hours.

Spicy Black Bean Chili

SERVINGS: 8 TO 10

PREPARATION TIME: 40 MINUTES (NEED COOKED BEANS)

COOKING TIME: 45 MINUTES

1 medium eggplant, cut into ½-inch cubes

1 cup vegetable broth (page 132) or water

2 medium onions, chopped

4 cloves garlic, minced

2 zucchini, chopped

1 red bell pepper, diced

1 yellow bell pepper, diced

One 28-ounce can Italian plum tomatoes, with juice

4 large ripe plum tomatoes, diced

½ cup chopped fresh parsley or cilantro

½ cup slivered fresh basil leaves

2 tablespoons chili powder

1 tablespoon ground cumin

2 teaspoons dried oregano

1 teaspoon freshly ground black pepper

¼ teaspoon crushed red pepper flakes

2 cups cooked black beans

1½ cups frozen corn kernels, thawed

½ cup chopped fresh dill

¼ cup fresh lemon juice

Preheat the broiler.

Place the eggplant on a nonstick baking sheet. Broil 8 inches from the heat source for about 5 minutes. Watch closely to make sure the eggplant doesn't burn. Remove from the broiler and set aside.

Place the broth in a large soup pot. Add the onions, garlic, zucchini, and peppers. Cook, stirring, for 10 minutes over medium heat.

Coarsely chop the canned tomatoes and add them to the pot, along with their juice. Add the fresh tomatoes, parsley, basil, and the rest of the seasonings. Stir in the eggplant, cover, and simmer over low heat for 20 minutes. Add the beans, corn, dill, and lemon juice, and cook for 10 minutes longer.

Three-Bean Chili

SERVINGS: 12
PREPARATION TIME: 25 MINUTES, PLUS 1 HOUR SOAKING TIME
COOKING TIME: 2 HOURS, 10 MINUTES

1 cup black beans
1 cup pinto beans
1 cup kidney beans
6½ cups water
1 cup chopped onion
1 cup chopped celery
1 green bell pepper, chopped
1 red bell pepper, chopped
3 cloves garlic, minced
¼ cup chili powder
½ tablespoon ground cumin
1 teaspoon ground oregano
¼ teaspoon crushed red pepper flakes
One 28-ounce can crushed tomatoes
One 4-ounce can chopped green chilies
Chopped scallion for garnish (optional)
Chopped fresh cilantro for garnish (optional)

Place the beans and 6 cups of the water in a large pot. Bring to a boil, boil for 2 minutes, and remove from the heat. Cover and let stand for 1 hour. Or, soak overnight in the water. Proceed as directed below, reducing cooking time by ½ hour.

In another pot, place the onion, celery, bell pepper, garlic, and the remaining ½ cup water. Sauté until the vegetables have softened slightly, about 6 minutes. Add the beans and their water, the chili powder, cumin, oregano, and red pepper. Bring to a boil, cover, reduce the heat, and cook for 1 hour. Stir in the tomatoes and chilies. Continue to cook for another hour. Garnish with chopped scallion and/or chopped cilantro before serving, if desired.

Note: This freezes well in a tightly covered container. Thaw overnight in the refrigerator and reheat on top of the stove or in the microwave.

Texas Crude

SERVINGS: 8 TO 10
PREPARATION TIME: 20 MINUTES, PLUS OVERNIGHT SOAKING
COOKING TIME: 2 TO 3 HOURS

(This recipe was sent by Fred Thornton of Dallas, Texas. I smiled when I read it because of the way it was written. I have left it pretty much the way Fred sent it in.) A sure-fire gusher of taste and a guaranteed well of "natural" gas. This find was brought in by an old vegetarian driller while trying to find a vegetarian subtitute for Texas Red. It didn't do the job but was so popular that we kept it pumping.

1 cup each black beans, red beans (small), lentils, and split peas
½ cup long-grain brown rice
One 14-ounce can stewed tomatoes
1 bay leaf

Dash crushed red pepper flakes
1 teaspoon chili powder
¼ cup brown sugar
1 stalk celery, diced
1 green bell pepper, diced
1 onion, diced

Soak the black and red beans separately, in water to cover, overnight. Pour off the water and pick out any rocks. Put the beans, lentils, peas, and rice in a large pot and add water to cover. Add the bay leaf, red pepper, chili powder, and brown sugar and bring to a boil. Add the remaining ingredients and reduce the heat to a simmer. Cook for a couple of hours, or until the black beans are no longer crunchy and the mixture looks like driller's mud (or until the old driller can't wait any longer, cuz it smells *so good*).

Variation: *Sunshiny Texas Crude.* The old driller's wife prefers to add a little Texas sunshine to this mix by putting in about 2 cups of frozen corn while it's coming to a boil.

Extra-Spicy Lentil Chili

SERVINGS: 6 TO 8
PREPARATION TIME: 15 MINUTES
COOKING TIME: 30 TO 35 MINUTES

Serve over brown rice, five-grain medley, or potatoes, or in a bowl by itself.

1 pound lentils
2 quarts vegetable broth (page 132) or water
2 cups diced onion
1 cup crushed tomatoes
¼ cup tomato paste
2 tablespoons chopped garlic
2 tablespoons balsamic vinegar
2 tablespoons fresh lime juice
1 tablespoon ground cumin
2 tablespoons chili powder
1 teaspoon cayenne (use less if you don't like your chili spicy)

Combine all of the ingredients in a large soup pot. Bring to a boil over high heat. Reduce the heat, cover, and simmer over medium-low heat until the lentils are tender, 30 to 35 minutes, adding more water or broth if needed for proper chili consistency.

Red-Hot Chili

SERVINGS: 6 TO 8

PREPARATION TIME: 20 MINUTES (NEED COOKED BEANS)

COOKING TIME: 1 HOUR

This chili is for those adventurous souls who want to wake up their taste buds. We like it very spicy, but you can reduce the amount of chili powder by one half if you prefer and then add more to taste.

One 28-ounce can whole tomatoes, chopped, with liquid

¾ cup bulghur

1 onion, coarsely chopped

½ cup water

3 stalks celery, coarsely chopped

2 carrots, scrubbed and chopped

5 tablespoons chili powder

2 to 4 cloves garlic, minced

1 tablespoon fresh lemon juice

1 teaspoon freshly ground pepper

1 teaspoon ground cumin

1 teaspoon dried basil

½ teaspoon dried oregano

1½ cups coarsely chopped green bell pepper

3 cups cooked red kidney beans

1½ cups cooked garbanzo beans

2 cups tomato juice

Drain the tomatoes, reserving the liquid. Bring 1 cup of the reserved liquid to a boil in a medium saucepan over medium heat. Remove the pan from the heat. Stir in the bulghur. Cover and let stand while cooking the vegetables.

Cook the onion in the water until translucent, stirring frequently. Add the drained tomatoes, celery, carrots, chili powder, garlic, lemon juice, pepper, cumin, basil, and oregano and cook until the vegetables are almost tender, stirring frequently (about 15 minutes). Add the green pepper and cook until tender, about 10 minutes. Add the soaked bulghur, the kidney and garbanzo beans, and the tomato juice. Mix well. Reduce the heat to low and simmer for 30 minutes, stirring occasionally. If it seems too thick, add the remaining tomato liquid or some water to thin it to the proper consistency.

Note: This can be prepared ahead. It reheats well over low heat.

CHAPTER 6

SALADS AND DRESSINGS

When you think of salads you generally think lettuce and maybe a few common vegetables, like carrots and cauliflower. But the traditional dinner salad has been all but replaced over the last few years. Every supermarket offers exotic selections of salad greens compared to a few years ago when your choice was head or leaf lettuce. This chapter is going to take you beyond the usual salad made of a few pieces of lettuce disguised by gobs of oil, mayonnaise, and sour cream, and beyond canned vegetables swimming in butter.

From now on you are going to think about rice, wild rice, bulghur, quinoa, couscous, corn, pasta, potatoes, and beans when you think of salad. Not only does the level of interest skyrocket by including these starchy vegetables, but the nutritional value becomes equivalent to a complete meal, and it follows that you may want to turn some of these salad recipes into your whole meal. But this time eating just a salad won't mean you'll be hungry an hour after you leave the table. Tomato Rice Salad, Fruited Wild Rice Salad, Tomato Tabouli Salad, Black Bean and Corn Salad, Zesty Red Potato Salad, and Potato-Vegetable Salad can serve as a main dish or a side salad.

If you want to emphasize the low-calorie qualities of salads, then make choices that are primarily made of green and yellow vegetables and fruits rather than starchy vegetables, like grains, potatoes, and beans. In this case try Green Papaya Salad, Thai Cabbage Salad, and Tomato Salad.

179

No longer are salad dressings limited to high-fat products. Healthy salad dressings—made without oil or animal products— are available at every market. They may have other ingredients, like preservatives, that will spur you on to make your own fresh dressings. In this chapter you will find some intriguing dressings, such as Honey-Tomato Dressing, Chili-Cilantro Dressing, Herbed Tofu Dressing or Dip, and Creamy Garlic Dressing. Dressings are not just for leafy greens; they also go well over broccoli, cauliflower, green beans, potatoes, and virtually any other vegetable.

Vegetable Salads

Red and Green Salad

SERVINGS: 4

PREPARATION TIME: 20 MINUTES

COOKING TIME: 35 MINUTES

This is a fresh, colorful, and tasty salad.

8 small fresh beets	¼ cup fresh-squeezed orange
1 medium-size firm, ripe	juice
pear	2 tablespoons raspberry-
1 teaspoon fresh lemon	flavored vinegar
juice	2 tablespoons water
2 bunches washed, trimmed	2 teaspoons ground
arugula	coriander
1 cup thinly sliced fennel	⅛ teaspoon freshly ground
bulb	pepper

Leave the roots and 1 inch of stem on the beets. Place them in a saucepan with water to cover. Bring to a boil, cover, reduce the heat, and simmer for 35 minutes, or until tender. Drain. Pour cold water over the beets and drain again. Trim off the roots and stems; rub off the skins. Cut each beet into eight wedges.

Halve the pear lengthwise; core and cut lengthwise into thin slices. Brush the cut sides with lemon juice. Set aside.

Line four salad plates with the arugula. Arrange the beet, pear, and fennel on the arugula.

Combine the remaining ingredients in a jar; cover and shake well. Drizzle a small amount of dressing over each salad.

Spring Salad

SERVINGS: 6 TO 8
PREPARATION TIME: 30 MINUTES

4 quarts (about 1 pound) salad greens (romaine, leaf lettuce, spinach, and/or radicchio), washed, drained, and torn
2 cups julienned jícama
1 cup snow peas, trimmed
½ cup thinly sliced red onion
2 oranges, peeled and sliced

1 small cucumber, thinly sliced
Oil-free dressing; try Strawberry Vinaigrette (page 207), Mango-Orange Dressing (page 208), or Chili-Cilantro Dressing (page 206)

Place the greens in a large salad bowl. Arrange the remaining ingredients over the greens. Pour the dressing over the salad and mix gently.

Cucumber-Dill Crunch

SERVINGS: MAKES 2 CUPS
PREPARATION TIME: 10 MINUTES
CHILLING TIME: 1 TO 2 HOURS

This is a very flavorful salad. We enjoy it as a snack in the middle of the afternoon. It's very refreshing on a hot day, and compliments potato dishes very nicely.

2 large cucumbers, thinly sliced
¼ cup finely chopped onion
1 clove garlic, sliced
1 teaspoon dill seeds
¼ cup fresh lemon juice

Toss all of the ingredients well. Cover and chill for 1 to 2 hours before serving.

Cabbage Slaw

SERVINGS: 4
PREPARATION TIME: 30 MINUTES
CHILLING TIME: 1 TO 2 HOURS

½ teaspoon salt (optional)
¼ teaspoon freshly ground black pepper
½ teaspoon dry mustard
1 teaspoon celery seeds
2 tablespoons sugar or honey
¼ cup chopped green bell pepper
1 tablespoon chopped red bell pepper or pimiento
½ teaspoon grated onion
⅓ cup white vinegar
3 cups finely chopped or shredded cabbage (not Savoy)

Place the salt, pepper, dry mustard, celery seeds, sugar, peppers, and onion in a large bowl. Mix well and stir in the vinegar. Add the cabbage and toss to mix well. Cover and chill for 1 to 2 hours before serving.

Variations: Tasty and colorful additions to this salad could include cut-up red apples, drained pineapple, halved green and seeded Tokay grapes, bananas, grated turnips, minced onions, grated raw carrots, celery, cucumbers, and dill seeds.

Pineapple Coleslaw

SERVINGS: 8
PREPARATION TIME: 30 MINUTES
COOKING TIME: 5 MINUTES
CHILLING TIME: 2 HOURS

2 cups water
3 tablespoons cornstarch
½ cup unsweetened pineapple juice
3 tablespoons fresh lemon juice
1 tablespoon vanilla extract

½ head green cabbage, shredded
⅛ head red cabbage, shredded
1 cup shredded carrot
1 cup crushed pineapple in its own juice, drained

In a saucepan combine the water and cornstarch. Bring to a boil and cook, stirring, until clear. Remove from the heat. Add the fruit juices and vanilla.

Combine the vegetables and pineapple. Add the dressing and mix well. Chill for 2 hours before serving.

Tomato Salad

SERVINGS: 6 TO 8
PREPARATION TIME: 15 MINUTES
CHILLING TIME: 1 HOUR

4 to 5 large vine-ripened
tomatoes
1 medium green bell
pepper
1 small sweet onion

1 to 2 teaspoons finely
chopped fresh basil
⅓ cup oil-free Italian
dressing

Coarsely chop the tomatoes, pepper, and onion. Place in a bowl; add the basil and dressing and mix well. Cover and chill for 1 hour or longer before serving.

Green Papaya Salad

SERVINGS: 6 TO 8
PREPARATION TIME: 30 MINUTES

When we lived in Hawaii, my favorite Thai restaurant made a wonderful Green Papaya Salad. After we moved to California, I couldn't find anything that came close, so I invented my own version.

2 cloves garlic
2 to 4 small red chili peppers
6½ tablespoons fresh lime
juice
4 tablespoons soy sauce

1 large green papaya (see
Note 1)
1 large tomato, sliced in
thin strips
Chinese cabbage leaves

Grind the garlic and chilies in a small food processor or with a mortar and pestle. Place the lime juice and soy sauce in a small jar. Add the pepper paste and shake well to mix. Set aside.

Peel the papaya and clean out the seeds. Shred the papaya in a food processor or with a hand grater. Pour the sauce over the papaya and mix well. Add the tomato strips and toss gently to mix. Serve on leaves of Chinese cabbage.

Notes: 1. Green papaya is unripe papaya. It is very firm with white flesh. It is not sweet, but tastes more like a very mild summer squash. You will probably be able to find it in an Asian grocery store.

2. This may be eaten like a regular salad with a fork, or rolled up in the cabbage leaves and eaten with your fingers.

Thai Vegetable Salad

SERVINGS: 6 TO 8
PREPARATION TIME: 30 MINUTES
CHILLING TIME: 1 TO 2 HOURS

This salad is also excellent with Savory Salad Dressing or Honey-Vinegar Dressing.

1½ cups shredded cabbage
1 cup shredded bok choy
1 cup mung bean
  sprouts
1 carrot, scrubbed and
  shredded

1 zucchini, cut in julienne
  strips
3 scallions, chopped
1 recipe Thai Dressing (page
  209)

Combine all of the vegetables in a large bowl. Pour the dressing over the vegetables and toss gently to mix well. Cover and chill for an hour or two before serving.

Thai Cabbage Salad

SERVINGS: 6 TO 8
PREPARATION TIME: 30 MINUTES

2 cloves garlic
2 to 4 small red chili
  peppers
6½ tablespoons fresh lime
  juice
4 tablespoons soy
  sauce

½ head green cabbage,
  shredded
½ head red cabbage,
  shredded
2 to 3 large carrots, scrubbed
  and grated
Lettuce leaves

Grind the garlic and chilies in a small food processor or with a mortar and pestle. Pour the lime juice and soy sauce into a small jar. Add the chili paste and shake well to mix. Set aside.

Place the shredded cabbage and carrot in a large bowl. Mix well. Pour the dressing over the vegetables and toss to mix. Serve on a bed of lettuce.

Zesty Red Potato Salad

SERVINGS: 6
PREPARATION TIME: 20 MINUTES (NEED COOKED POTATOES)
COOKING TIME: 4 MINUTES

1 cup snow peas, trimmed
4 cups sliced boiled red
  potatoes
⅓ cup sliced radish
¼ cup chopped scallion

⅔ cup nonfat dressing, such
  as Creamy Garlic (page
  210), Honey-Vinegar (page
  207), or a bottled dressing

Steam the snow peas over 1 inch of boiling water for about 4 minutes. Combine with the remaining ingredients and toss lightly to mix. Serve at once.

Potato Salad

SERVINGS: 8 TO 10
PREPARATION TIME: 30 MINUTES
COOKING TIME: 30 TO 40 MINUTES
CHILLING TIME: 2 HOURS

15 medium salad potatoes
4 to 6 scallions, chopped
1 stalk celery, chopped

1 small carrot, scrubbed
and grated
⅓ cucumber, chopped

DRESSING

1 pound soft tofu
1 to 2 tablespoons cider
vinegar
1 tablespoon fresh lemon
juice
2 tablespoons prepared
mustard

1½ teaspoons parsley
flakes
½ teaspoon honey
¼ teaspoon dried dill

Boil the potatoes until they are tender but still firm, about 30 minutes. Cool. Peel them if you wish, and cut into pieces. Combine all of the vegetables in a large bowl.

To make the dressing, combine the tofu and remaining ingredients in a blender or food processor and process until smooth. Pour over the vegetables and mix well. Chill for at least 2 hours before serving.

Potato-Vegetable Salad

SERVINGS: 8 TO 10
PREPARATION TIME: 30 MINUTES (NEED COOKED POTATOES)
COOKING TIME: 10 MINUTES
CHILLING TIME: 1 HOUR

4 red potatoes, boiled until tender
2 carrots, scrubbed and sliced
½ pound green beans, cut into 1-inch pieces
2 cups cauliflower florets
1 zucchini, cut lengthwise in half and sliced

1 cucumber, peeled and chopped
1 bunch scallions, chopped
¼ cup chopped fresh cilantro
Double recipe Creamy Garlic Dressing (page 210)

Chop the potatoes and place them in a large bowl. Steam the carrots, beans, cauliflower, and zucchini until just tender, about 10 minutes. Add to the potatoes along with the cucumber, scallions, and cilantro. Toss with the dressing and chill for an hour or more. Mix again before serving.

Pasta Salads

Garden Pasta Salad

SERVINGS: 8 TO 10
PREPARATION TIME: 30 MINUTES
COOKING TIME: 10 MINUTES
CHILLING TIME: 2 HOURS

4 quarts water
One 10- to 12-ounce
   package tricolor rotini
   pasta
1 cup chopped broccoli
1 cup chopped
   cauliflower
1 cup snow peas,
   trimmed
1 cup sliced mushrooms

3 scallions, thinly sliced
One 2-ounce jar chopped
   pimientos, drained
¾ cup cherry tomatoes,
   cut in half
¾ to 1 cup oil-free Italian
   dressing
Freshly ground black
   pepper to taste

Bring the water to a boil and add the pasta. Return to boiling and cook, uncovered, for 6 minutes. Drain. Rinse under cool water and set aside.

Place the broccoli, cauliflower, and snow peas in a steamer basket. Steam over boiling water for 4 to 5 minutes, until tender-crisp.

Combine all of the ingredients in a large bowl. Toss to mix well. Refrigerate for at least 2 hours before serving.

Pesto Pasta Salad

SERVINGS: 8

PREPARATION TIME: 30 MINUTES (NEED COOKED PASTA)

COOKING TIME: 2 TO 3 MINUTES

1 pound fresh spinach
1 cup fresh basil leaves
3 to 4 cloves garlic
½ cup low-fat soy milk
½ cup oil-free Italian
   dressing
¼ cup chopped fresh
   parsley
3 tablespoons onion
   powder
2 tablespoons soy sauce

4 cups cooked rotelli (or
   other shape) pasta
1 cup sliced mushrooms
1 cup diced carrot
1 cup diced cucumber
1 cup cherry tomatoes,
   cut in half
½ cup diced yellow or
   green bell pepper, or a
   combination

Trim and wash the spinach. Place it in a saucepan with some water clinging to the leaves. Cover and cook over medium heat until wilted, about 2 to 3 minutes. Drain off the water. Set aside.

Place the basil, garlic, soy milk, dressing, parsley, onion powder, and soy sauce in a blender or food processor. Add the spinach and process until smooth.

Place the remaining ingredients in a large bowl. Add the blended dressing and toss to mix.

Rotini Salad

SERVINGS: 4 TO 6

PREPARATION TIME: 20 MINUTES

COOKING TIME: 6 TO 7 MINUTES

CHILLING TIME: 1 TO 2 HOURS

4 quarts water
½ pound rotini

1 cup each chopped red and
   yellow bell pepper

½ small red onion, chopped
¼ pound snow peas, trimmed
2 tablespoons fresh lemon juice

1 tablespoon soy sauce
1 clove garlic, minced
Dash ground ginger

Bring the water to a boil and add the rotini. Cook until just tender, 6 to 7 minutes. Drain. Add the peppers, onion, and snow peas. In a small bowl, blend the lemon juice, soy sauce, garlic, and ginger. Toss with the rotini mixture. Chill for 1 to 2 hours before serving.

Summer Pasta Salad

SERVINGS: 8
PREPARATION TIME: 30 MINUTES
COOKING TIME: 16 TO 20 MINUTES

4 quarts water
1 pound pasta
2 cups broccoli florets
1 cup slivered carrot
20 snow peas, trimmed
1 bunch scallions, cut into 1-inch pieces
1 pint cherry tomatoes, cut in half

½ cup sliced fresh basil, loosely packed
½ cup Creamy Garlic Dressing (page 210), Honey-Vinegar Dressing (page 207), or Savory Salad Dressing (page 209)
½ cup grated soy Parmesan cheese (optional)

Bring the water to a boil. Add the pasta and cook until just tender, about 8 to 10 minutes. Drain well.

Place the broccoli and carrot in a large saucepan with about ¼ cup water. Cover and cook over medium heat for 3 to 4 minutes. Add the snow peas and cook for another 3 to 4 minutes. Add the scallions and cook for another 2 minutes.

Remove from the heat, drain, and place in a large bowl. Add the tomatoes, basil, cooked pasta, and the dressing of your choice. Toss to mix well. Add the soy Parmesan cheese, if desired, and toss again. Serve warm or cold.

Wild Rice and Pasta Salad

SERVINGS: 6

PREPARATION TIME: 20 MINUTES (NEED COOKED RICE AND PASTA)

CHILLING TIME: 4 HOURS

⅓ cup dry-packed sun-dried tomatoes

1 cup cooked wild rice

1 cup cooked orzo

½ medium red or green bell pepper, chopped

½ cup chopped mushrooms

1 tablespoon drained capers

⅓ cup balsamic vinegar

1 tablespoon soy sauce

2 tablespoons water

2 tablespoons chopped fresh basil

1 tablespoon finely chopped shallot or scallion

2 cloves garlic, minced

½ teaspoon freshly ground pepper

Soften the tomatoes by soaking them in boiling water for 2 minutes. Drain and chop. In a large mixing bowl, combine the rice, orzo, pepper, mushrooms, tomatoes, and capers; set aside. Combine the remaining ingredients in a jar with a tight-fitting lid. Cover and shake well. Pour over the rice mixture and toss to coat. Cover and chill for at least 4 hours before serving.

Grain and Bean Salads

Tomato-Rice Salad

SERVINGS: 6

PREPARATION TIME: 25 MINUTES (NEED COOKED RICE AND BARLEY)

CHILLING TIME: 2 HOURS

This salad is also excellent stuffed into six hollowed-out tomatoes.

1 tablespoon fresh lemon juice
½ teaspoon honey
¼ teaspoon garlic powder
¼ teaspoon dried dill
1½ cups cooked brown rice
½ cup cooked barley
2 tomatoes, diced

⅓ cup diced red onion
¼ cup diced cucumber
¼ cup sliced carrot
¼ cup diced celery
¼ cup diced green bell pepper
Fresh parsley for garnish

Combine the lemon juice, honey, garlic powder, and dill in a large bowl. Add all of the remaining ingredients, except the parsley, and toss well to coat. Chill for at least 2 hours. Garnish with parsley before serving.

Curried Rice Salad

SERVINGS: 8
PREPARATION TIME: 20 MINUTES
COOKING TIME: 1 HOUR

1 onion, chopped
1 clove garlic, minced
3¼ cups water
1½ cups long-grain brown
   rice

1 tablespoon curry powder
⅛ teaspoon white pepper
2 cups chopped broccoli
1 bunch scallions, chopped
2 tomatoes, chopped

SAUCE

1 tablespoon water
1 tablespoon low-sodium
   soy sauce

1 tablespoon white-wine
   vinegar

Place the onion and garlic in a saucepan with ¼ cup of the water. Cook, stirring, until the onion softens slightly, about 5 minutes. Add the rice, the remaining 3 cups water, the curry powder, and the pepper. Stir. Bring to a boil, reduce the heat to low, cover, and simmer for 45 minutes.

Meanwhile, cook the broccoli in a small amount of water, stirring occasionally, until tender-crisp, about 5 minutes. Remove from the heat, drain, and set aside.

After the rice has cooked for 45 minutes, remove from the heat and let stand for 15 minutes without stirring. Then add the broccoli, scallions, and tomatoes. Toss gently. Combine the sauce ingredients. Pour over the rice and vegetables. Mix well. Serve warm or cold.

Fruited Wild Rice Salad

SERVINGS: 6 TO 8
PREPARATION TIME: 20 MINUTES
COOKING TIME: 1 HOUR
CHILLING TIME: 1 HOUR OR LONGER

1 cup wild rice
4 cups water
2 tablespoons soy sauce
1 tablespoon mustard seeds
1 tablespoon coriander seeds
1 teaspoon dried thyme
½ teaspoon ground allspice
½ cup chopped dates

½ cup chopped dried
unsulphured apricots
½ cup chopped fresh parsley
¼ cup chopped scallion
¼ cup fresh lemon juice
Freshly ground pepper to
taste

Rinse the rice and place it in a large saucepan. Add the water, soy sauce, and spices. Bring to a boil, reduce the heat, cover, and simmer until the rice is tender, about 50 minutes. Drain and reserve the liquid. Set aside.

Combine the remaining ingredients in a large bowl. Add the rice and mix well. Add enough of the reserved liquid to make the salad as moist as you would like. Add more freshly ground pepper to taste.

Two-Bean and Rice Salad

SERVINGS: 6 TO 8
PREPARATION TIME: 20 MINUTES (NEED COOKED RICE)
CHILLING TIME: 2 HOURS OR LONGER

3 cups cooked brown rice
One 15-ounce can pinto
beans, rinsed and
drained
One 15-ounce can black
beans, rinsed and
drained
One 10-ounce package frozen
green peas, thawed

1 cup sliced celery
1 medium red onion,
chopped
One 7-ounce can chopped
green chilies
¼ cup chopped fresh
cilantro or parsley
One 8-ounce jar oil-free
Italian dressing

Combine all of the ingredients in a large bowl. Toss gently until
well mixed. Cover and chill for at least 2 hours before serving.

Vegetable-Barley Salad

SERVINGS: 8
PREPARATION TIME: 20 MINUTES
COOKING TIME: 30 MINUTES
CHILLING TIME: 2 HOURS OR LONGER

½ cup barley
2 cups water
2 cups frozen corn kernels,
thawed
1 cup frozen green peas,
thawed

1 tomato, chopped
¼ cup chopped scallion
1 tablespoon chopped fresh
basil or oregano

DRESSING

2 tablespoons cider vinegar
2 tablespoons water
2 tablespoons soy sauce

1 teaspoon Dijon mustard
¼ teaspoon freshly ground
pepper

Place the barley and water in a small saucepan. Cover and cook over low heat until the barley is tender, about 30 minutes. Drain and set aside.

Combine the corn, peas, tomato, scallion, and fresh herbs in a bowl. Add the barley and toss to mix.

In a small jar or bowl, mix the dressing ingredients together thoroughly. Pour the dressing over the salad and mix well. For best flavor, cover and chill for at least 2 hours before serving.

Couscous Salad

SERVINGS: 10 TO 12
PREPARATION TIME: 30 MINUTES
CHILLING TIME: 4 TO 6 HOURS

One 10-ounce package
 couscous
2 cups water
1 large carrot, scrubbed
 and shredded
1 green bell pepper,
 chopped
1 zucchini, cut in half
 lengthwise, then sliced

1 yellow summer squash,
 cut in half lengthwise,
 then sliced
1 cup cherry tomatoes, cut
 in half
1 cup oil-free salad
 dressing

Place the couscous in a large casserole. Boil the water and pour over the couscous. Cover and let rest for 15 minutes.

Prepare the vegetables as directed. Add to the couscous. Mix well. Add the dressing, toss, cover, and chill for 4 to 6 hours before serving.

Tabouli

SERVINGS: 6 TO 8
PREPARATION TIME: 15 MINUTES
SOAKING TIME: 1 HOUR
CHILLING TIME: 2 HOURS OR LONGER

1 cup bulghur	2 teaspoons minced garlic
2 cups boiling water	1 teaspoon freshly ground
½ cup fresh lemon juice	black pepper
½ cup chopped fresh mint	2 tomatoes, chopped
1 cup chopped fresh parsley	1 cup cooked garbanzo
½ cup chopped scallion	beans

Put the bulghur in a mixing bowl. Pour the boiling water over the bulghur. Cover with a towel and let stand for 1 hour. After 1 hour, the excess water must be removed. The easiest way to do this is to pour the bulghur and the water into a fine mesh strainer. Let the water drain off, pressing the bulghur with your hands to remove as much of the excess water as possible. Place the drained bulghur in a bowl. Add the remaining ingredients. Toss well to mix. Cover and refrigerate for at least 2 hours to allow the flavors to blend.

Barley Salad

SERVINGS: 6 TO 8
PREPARATION TIME: 30 MINUTES
COOKING TIME: 35 MINUTES
CHILLING TIME: 2 HOURS OR LONGER

1 cup barley	¼ cup chopped fresh mint
2 quarts water	¼ cup chopped fresh cilantro
1 tomato, chopped	¼ cup fresh lemon juice
1 cup chopped cucumber	⅛ teaspoon garlic powder
½ cup chopped fresh parsley	Dash cayenne (optional)

Place the barley in a large nonstick frying pan. Toast over medium heat, stirring constantly, until golden, 3 to 4 minutes. Place the water in a large saucepan. Bring to a boil, add the toasted barley, cover, reduce the heat, and simmer for 30 minutes. Drain. Combine the cooked barley with the remaining ingredients. Cover and refrigerate for at least 2 hours before serving.

Quinoa Salad

SERVINGS: 8 TO 10
PREPARATION TIME: 15 MINUTES
COOKING TIME: 15 MINUTES
CHILLING TIME: 2 HOURS OR LONGER

Quinoa (pronounced keen-wa) is a high-protein grain. It was popular many years ago, and has just recently become available again. Uncooked, it looks somewhat like toasted sesame seeds. After cooking, it becomes translucent. Most natural-food stores carry quinoa.

1½ cups quinoa
3 cups water
1 green bell pepper, chopped
1 red bell pepper, chopped
¼ cup chopped scallion
¼ cup chopped red onion

¼ cup finely chopped fresh dill, cilantro, or parsley
1 recipe Savory Salad Dressing (page 209) or Honey-Vinegar Dressing (page 207)
Freshly ground pepper to taste

Rinse the quinoa well before cooking to remove its slightly bitter coating. Place the quinoa and water in a saucepan. Bring to a boil, cover, reduce the heat, and simmer for about 15 minutes, or until the liquid is absorbed.

Combine the chopped vegetables in a bowl, including the fresh chopped herb of your choice. Mix well. Add the cooked quinoa. Toss gently and add dressing of your choice. Toss again and add pepper to taste. Cover and chill for at least 2 hours before serving.

Tomato Tabouli Salad

SERVINGS: 4
PREPARATION TIME: 15 MINUTES, PLUS 1 HOUR SOAKING TIME
CHILLING TIME: 4 HOURS

½ cup bulghur
1 cup boiling water
One 14-ounce can stewed
  tomatoes
½ cup chopped fresh
  parsley
¼ cup chopped fresh mint

¼ cup currants or raisins
¼ cup fresh lemon juice
1 clove garlic, crushed
1 teaspoon curry powder
¼ teaspoon ground cumin
¼ teaspoon ground
  cinnamon

Place the bulghur in a bowl and pour the boiling water over it. Stir, cover, and let stand for 1 hour. Drain according to the directions on page 82.

Drain the tomatoes, reserving ¼ cup of juice. Chop the tomatoes, then combine with the parsley, mint, and currants or raisins. Add the drained bulghur and mix well.

Combine the reserved tomato juice with the remaining ingredients. Pour over the bulghur mixture and toss to mix. Refrigerate for 4 hours before serving.

Black Bean and Corn Salad

SERVINGS: 6 TO 8
PREPARATION TIME: 20 MINUTES
CHILLING TIME: 1 HOUR OR LONGER

Two 15-ounce cans black
  beans, rinsed and
  drained
2 cups frozen corn
  kernels, thawed

1 red or green bell
  pepper, chopped
One 4-ounce can chopped
  green chilies

1 recipe Savory Salad
Dressing (page 209)
1 pint cherry tomatoes,
cut in half

3 to 4 scallions, chopped
¼ cup chopped fresh
cilantro

In a large casserole dish, combine the beans, corn, pepper, and chilies. Add the dressing and mix well. Cover and chill for at least 1 hour. Before serving, add the remaining ingredients and toss to mix well.

Black Bean Salad

SERVINGS: 2
PREPARATION TIME: 15 MINUTES
CHILLING TIME: 2 HOURS

This recipe can easily be doubled, but we often make just enough for a light, satisfying lunch.

One 16-ounce can black
beans, rinsed and
drained
1 green bell pepper, diced
½ cup diced tomato

2 scallions, sliced
4 teaspoons fresh lemon
juice
⅛ teaspoon freshly ground
black pepper

Combine the beans with the vegetables. Mix the lemon juice and black pepper. Pour the dressing over the beans and vegetables. Mix well. Chill for 2 hours before serving.

Spicy Three-Bean Salad

SERVINGS: 6 TO 8

PREPARATION TIME: 15 MINUTES   CHILLING TIME: 1 HOUR OR LONGER

One 15-ounce can black beans, rinsed and drained

One 15-ounce can garbanzo beans, rinsed and drained

One 15-ounce can kidney beans, rinsed and drained

1 small red onion, thinly sliced

2 stalks celery, thinly sliced

1 tomato, chopped

1 cup oil-free salsa

Juice of 1 lime

1 teaspoon chili powder (optional)

Freshly ground pepper to taste

Combine the beans and vegetables in a large bowl. Place the salsa in a small bowl or jar. Add the lime juice, the chili powder, if desired, and pepper. Mix well.

Pour the salsa mixture over the beans. Toss to mix well. Cover and refrigerate for at least 1 hour to allow the flavors to blend.

Marinated Lentil Salad

SERVINGS: 4 TO 6

PREPARATION TIME: 30 MINUTES

COOKING TIME: 5 MINUTES   CHILLING TIME: 1 HOUR OR LONGER

½ pound lentils

2 quarts water

1 bay leaf

1 whole clove garlic, peeled

1 bunch scallions, thinly sliced

1 cup finely chopped red or green bell pepper

½ cup finely chopped fresh parsley

½ cup shredded carrot

4 tablespoons fresh lemon juice

½ tablespoon soy sauce

1 teaspoon Dijon mustard

½ teaspoon freshly ground black pepper

Clean the lentils and place them in a large pot. Add the water, bay leaf, and garlic. Heat to boiling, turn the heat off, and let stand for 30 minutes. Drain. Remove the bay leaf and garlic. Place the lentils in a large bowl.

Add the scallion, bell pepper, parsley, and carrot. Mix well.

Combine the remaining ingredients in a small bowl. Blend thoroughly. Pour over the lentil mixture and toss well. Chill for at least 1 hour before serving.

Variation: This is also delicious made with fresh dill instead of, or in addition to, the parsley. Use 1 to 2 tablespoons, minced.

Bean and Rice Salad

SERVINGS: 10 TO 12

PREPARATION TIME: 30 MINUTES (NEED COOKED RICE)

CHILLING TIME: 2 HOURS OR LONGER

3 cups cooked brown rice

One 15-ounce can black beans, rinsed and drained

One 15-ounce can pinto beans, rinsed and drained

1 red onion, chopped

2 stalks celery, sliced

1 red or green bell pepper, chopped

One 4-ounce can chopped green chilies

1 cup frozen corn kernels, thawed

1 cup frozen green peas, thawed

¼ cup chopped fresh parsley or cilantro

1 recipe Chili-Cilantro Dressing (page 206), Savory Salad Dressing (page 209), or Creamy Garlic Dressing (page 210), or about ⅔ cup of your favorite oil-free dressing

Combine all of the ingredients in a large bowl and mix well. Cover and refrigerate for at least 2 hours to allow the flavors to blend.

White Bean Salad

SERVINGS: 4

PREPARATION TIME: 10 MINUTES (PLUS OVERNIGHT SOAKING)

COOKING TIME: 1½ HOURS

CHILLING TIME: 4 HOURS

This recipe can easily be doubled and it is a good dish to take to a potluck dinner.

1 cup Great Northern beans	1 bay leaf
1 quart water	⅓ cup fresh lemon juice
1 onion, chopped	½ teaspoon ground cumin
2 cloves garlic, pressed	

GARNISHES

2 tomatoes, chopped	¼ cup finely chopped fresh
6 scallions, chopped	parsley or cilantro

Soak the beans overnight in enough water to cover plus 2 inches.

Drain the beans. Place them in a pot with the 1 quart water, onion, garlic, and bay leaf. Bring to a boil, reduce the heat, cover, and cook over low heat for 1½ hours, or until the beans are tender.

Drain the beans, reserving the cooking liquid. Place the beans in a bowl, discarding the bay leaf, and set aside.

In a separate bowl, combine ⅓ cup of the bean cooking liquid, the lemon juice, and the cumin. Pour over the beans and toss to coat. Refrigerate for at least 4 hours before serving. Just before serving, toss again with the garnishes.

Spicy Mexican Bean Salad

SERVINGS: 8 TO 10
PREPARATION TIME: 30 MINUTES (NEEDS COOKED BEANS)
COOKING TIME: 4 TO 5 MINUTES
CHILLING TIME: 1 TO 2 HOURS

1 red onion, sliced
¼ cup water
1 tablespoon chili powder
2 cups cooked green beans
One 15-ounce can black beans, drained and rinsed
One 15-ounce can red kidney beans, drained and rinsed

One 15-ounce can white beans, drained and rinsed
1½ cups frozen corn kernels, thawed
2 tablespoons chopped fresh cilantro or parsley
½ cup Chili-Cilantro Dressing (page 206), Savory Salad Dressing (page 209), or oil-free dressing of your choice

Place the onion in a saucepan with the water. Cook gently until the onion is soft and separated into rings, 4 to 5 minutes. Add the chili powder and stir until well mixed. Remove from the heat.

Combine all of the ingredients in a large bowl and toss to mix well. Cover and chill for 1 to 2 hours to allow the flavors to blend.

Kidney Bean Salad

SERVINGS: 8

PREPARATION TIME: 10 MINUTES (NEED COOKED BEANS AND PREPARED TOFU
CREAM CHEESE)

CHILLING TIME: 2 HOURS

*Try this stuffed into pita bread with lettuce leaves and topped with salsa
or your favorite oil-free dressing.*

3 cups cooked kidney beans
¼ cup chopped green bell
  pepper

¼ cup chopped red onion
¾ cup Tofu Cream Cheese
  (page 122)

Combine all of the ingredients and mix well. Chill for 2 hours to allow the flavors to blend.

Dressings

Chili-Cilantro Dressing

SERVINGS: MAKES ¾ CUP

PREPARATION TIME: 10 MINUTES

One 4-ounce can chopped
  green chilies
¼ cup chopped fresh
  cilantro
¼ cup water

¼ cup fresh lime juice
1 to 2 cloves garlic
2 teaspoons honey
Freshly ground pepper
to taste

Place all of the ingredients in a food processor or blender. Process
until smooth.

Strawberry Vinaigrette

SERVINGS: MAKES 1 CUP
PREPARATION TIME: 10 MINUTES

1 cup strawberries, fresh or
 frozen
2 tablespoons red-wine
 vinegar

1 teaspoon honey or barley
 malt
Freshly ground pepper to
 taste

Combine all of the ingredients in a food processor or blender. Process until smooth.

Honey-Vinegar Dressing

SERVINGS: MAKES ⅔ CUP
PREPARATION TIME: 5 MINUTES

¼ cup balsamic vinegar
¼ cup rice vinegar
2½ tablespoons honey
1½ tablespoons Dijon
 mustard

Freshly ground pepper to
 taste

Place all of the ingredients in a jar. Cover and shake until well blended.

Honey-Tomato Dressing

SERVINGS: MAKES ⅔ CUP
PREPARATION TIME: 5 MINUTES

¼ cup honey
2 tablespoons catsup
2 tablespoons cider vinegar

2 tablespoons water
½ teaspoon Worcestershire
  sauce

Place all of the ingredients in a jar. Cover and shake until well blended.

Mango-Orange Dressing

SERVINGS: MAKES ¾ CUP
PREPARATION TIME: 10 MINUTES

1 medium mango, peeled
  and cut into chunks
½ cup fresh-squeezed orange
  juice

1 clove garlic, crushed
1 teaspoon soy sauce
¼ teaspoon curry powder

Place all of the ingredients in a food processor or blender. Process until smooth.

Savory Salad Dressing

SERVINGS: MAKES ⅔ CUP
PREPARATION TIME: 5 MINUTES

This dressing is especially good on grain-based salads.

1 teaspoon Dijon mustard
¼ cup red-wine vinegar
¼ cup water

¼ cup soy sauce
Several dashes Tabasco

Place all of the ingredients in a jar. Cover and shake until well blended.

Thai Dressing

SERVINGS: MAKES ⅔ CUP
PREPARATION TIME: 10 MINUTES
COOKING TIME: 5 MINUTES

½ cup water
3 tablespoons white-wine vinegar
1 tablespoon soy sauce
2 teaspoons honey
1½ teaspoons cornstarch

1 tablespoon peanut butter
1 tablespoon chopped fresh cilantro
1 clove garlic, crushed
¼ teaspoon crushed red pepper flakes

Combine the water, vinegar, soy sauce, honey, and cornstarch in a saucepan. Bring to a boil and cook, stirring constantly, until the mixture thickens. Remove from the heat. Stir in the peanut butter until smooth. Add the remaining ingredients and stir until well combined.

Herbed Tofu Dressing or Dip

SERVINGS: MAKES 2 CUPS
PREPARATION TIME: 10 MINUTES

This is one of my favorite salad dressings, and it also makes an excellent dip for vegetables.

⅔ cup water
2 cups packed fresh parsley
1 cup packed fresh cilantro leaves
½ to 1 pound tofu, crumbled (see Note)

4 cloves garlic
2 tablespoons white vinegar
1 tablespoon soy sauce

Place the water, parsley, and cilantro in a blender. Process until liquefied. Add the remaining ingredients and process until smooth.

Note: Use ½ pound of tofu for a thin dressing and up to 1 pound of tofu to make a thicker dip.

Creamy Garlic Dressing

SERVINGS: MAKES ⅔ CUP
PREPARATION TIME: 10 MINUTES

1 to 2 cloves garlic, crushed
¼ pound firm tofu, drained
¼ cup water
3 tablespoons fresh lemon juice
1 tablespoon soy sauce

1 tablespoon tahini
1 tablespoon chopped fresh dill
1 teaspoon honey
Freshly ground pepper to taste

Place all of the ingredients in a food processor or blender. Process until smooth and creamy.

Caesar Salad Dressing

SERVINGS: MAKES 3 CUPS
PREPARATION TIME: 10 MINUTES

This is a much healthier alternative to the traditional Caesar salad dressing, which is made with eggs and oil. It keeps well in the refrigerator for up to 1 week in a covered container.

To serve: Place about ¾ cup of the dressing in a large salad bowl. Add about 12 cups washed, drained, and torn romaine lettuce. Toss to coat. Add croutons made from Easy No-Fat Garlic Bread, if desired.

1 pound soft tofu
¼ cup fresh lemon juice
¼ cup soy sauce
2 tablespoons red-wine vinegar
3 tablespoons grated soy Parmesan cheese

2 cloves garlic, crushed
1 tablespoon Dijon mustard
Freshly ground pepper to taste
1 tablespoon drained capers

Place all of the ingredients, except the capers, in a blender or food processor and process until smooth. Add the capers. Refrigerate until ready to use.

Thousand Island Tofu Dressing

SERVINGS: MAKES 1 QUART
PREPARATION TIME: 10 MINUTES

**Three 10-ounce packages
firm tofu**
1 cup catsup
**1 tablespoon soy
sauce**

**2 tablespoons cider
vinegar**
**1 tablespoon (or less)
Mrs. Dash or other salt
substitute**

Place all of the ingredients in a food processor or blender and process until silky. This keeps well in the refrigerator for 1 week in a covered container.

Variation: For a chunky, zesty addition, stir in ½ cup of pickle relish. Do not blend.

CHAPTER 7

MAIN DISHES

Any one recipe in this chapter is usually enough to be satisfying for hunger and palate—consider it a whole meal. Serving sizes for these main-dish recipes may seem large, especially if you're eating alone or with one other person. We suggest you make the recipe as is and then freeze or refrigerate what's left over. It can be eaten as a main dish or be served as a side dish a second day. You may also find the leftovers a useful component of a new meal, such as stuffing for pita bread or topping for baked potatoes.

Some of the recipes are fast and easy, such as Quick Bulghur with Pasta, Quick Sautéed Spiced Vegetables with Rice, and Black Bean Burritos. Others, such as Thai Vegetable Curry, Mu Shu Vegetables, Seitan Bourguignon, and Pasta Primavera take a little extra time, offering a challenge to the more dedicated cook. But the results are worth the effort.

Main Dish Vegetables

Mushrooms McDougall

SERVINGS: 4 TO 8, DEPENDING ON USE
PREPARATION TIME: 15 MINUTES
COOKING TIME: 15 MINUTES

Serve rolled up in a burrito shell with fresh salsa; use on top of beans in a Mexican-style burrito; or serve on top of whole-wheat toast or baked potatoes. Invent your own favorite base. This is wonderful on almost anything!

¼ cup water
1½ pounds mushrooms, sliced
1 bunch scallions, chopped
2 cloves garlic, minced
One 4-ounce can chopped green chilies

2 tablespoons fresh lemon juice
¼ cup sherry or apple juice
½ teaspoon Worcestershire sauce
Freshly ground pepper to taste

Place the water in a large pan or wok. Bring to a boil; add the mushrooms, scallions, garlic, and chilies. Cook, stirring, for a minute or two, then add the remaining ingredients. Cook over medium heat, stirring frequently, until all of the liquid has been absorbed, 10 to 12 minutes.

Mushroom Stroganoff

SERVINGS: 6 TO 8
PREPARATION TIME: 20 MINUTES
COOKING TIME: 30 MINUTES

Serve over pasta or baked potatoes.

1 large onion, chopped
1 pound mushrooms, sliced
1 cup soy milk
1 cup vegetable broth (page 132) or water
2 tablespoons soy sauce
2 tablespoons sherry or apple juice

Dash cayenne
2 cups sliced seitan or firm tofu
2 tablespoons cornstarch or arrowroot, mixed with ⅓ cup cold water

Sauté the onion in a small amount of water for 2 to 3 minutes. Add the mushrooms and sauté until the mushrooms are slightly limp. Add the soy milk, broth, soy sauce, sherry (or apple juice), and cayenne. Stir well. Add the seitan or tofu. Mix. Cover and cook over low heat for 20 minutes. Add the cornstarch or arrowroot mixture to the pan and stir until thickened.

This will keep in the refrigerator up to a week in a covered container. *Do not freeze.*

Sweet and Sour Vegetables

SERVINGS: 6

PREPARATION TIME: 30 MINUTES

COOKING TIME: 15 MINUTES

Serve over rice or other whole grains.

One 20-ounce can pineapple chunks in their own juice

1 onion, cut in wedges

1 bunch scallions, cut into 1-inch pieces

1 large green bell pepper, cut into 1-inch pieces

1 cup sliced carrots

4 cups chopped broccoli

1 cup water

2 cloves garlic, crushed

1 teaspoon grated fresh ginger

SAUCE

1 cup unsweetened pineapple juice

⅓ cup brown sugar

¼ cup cider vinegar

2½ tablespoons soy sauce

2 tablespoons cornstarch

Drain the pineapple, reserve the juice, and set aside.

Place the vegetables, except the broccoli, in a large pot or wok with ½ cup of the water and the garlic and ginger. Sauté for 5 minutes. Add the broccoli and the remaining ½ cup water. Stir, then cover and cook over low heat for 5 minutes.

Combine the sauce ingredients in a separate bowl.

Stir in the pineapple chunks and the sauce mixture. Cook, stirring until thickened.

Sweet and Tangy Vegetables

SERVINGS: 6 TO 8
PREPARATION TIME: 30 MINUTES
COOKING TIME: 15 MINUTES

Serve as is or over whole grains, pasta, or potatoes.

SAUCE

1½ cups unsweetened apple juice
¼ cup soy sauce
1 tablespoon cider vinegar
1 tablespoon honey

2 teaspoons grated fresh ginger
2 teaspoons minced garlic
2½ tablespoons cornstarch

1 cup water
1 onion, coarsely chopped
1 cup sliced carrots

2 cups broccoli florets
2 cups cauliflower florets
2 cups sliced mushrooms

Combine the sauce ingredients and set aside.

Place the water and all of the vegetables except the mushrooms in a pot or wok. Cover and cook over medium heat for 10 minutes. Add the mushrooms. Stir and cook for an additional 5 minutes. Then stir in the sauce mixture. Cook, stirring, until thickened.

Quick Swiss Chard Tart

SERVINGS: MAKES ONE 10-INCH TART
PREPARATION TIME: 30 MINUTES
RISING TIME: 1 HOUR
COOKING TIME: 30 TO 45 MINUTES

CRUST

1 cup warm water
1 tablespoon active dry yeast
⅔ cup whole-wheat pastry
flour

⅓ cup cornmeal
½ teaspoon honey
½ teaspoon salt

FILLING

1 bunch Swiss chard,
washed and chopped
1 onion, sliced
1 carrot, scrubbed and grated

1 clove garlic, chopped
¼ cup water
1 tablespoon soy sauce

Mix the crust ingredients together in a large bowl to make a thick sponge. Stir with a spoon briskly about fifty times. Cover the bowl and place in a warm place for about ½ hour, or until the batter is bubbly. Add enough additional pastry flour to make a soft, sticky dough. Pour into a 10-inch pie plate or baking pan that has been oiled very lightly. Sprinkle a little flour on top of the dough so that you can pat the dough in the pan and up the edges about 1½ inches. Let rise ½ hour in a warm place.

Preheat the oven to 375°F.

Sauté the vegetables in the water and soy sauce until just barely tender. Fill the tart crust and bake for 30 to 45 minutes, or until the crust is lightly browned.

Broccoli with "Cheese" Sauce

SERVINGS: 6
PREPARATION TIME: 30 MINUTES
COOKING TIME: 25 MINUTES

Serve by itself or over baked potatoes.

SAUCE

¾ cup peeled, chopped potato
4 cups water
One 7-ounce jar chopped pimientos
½ cup brewer's yeast

⅓ cup cornstarch
¼ cup fresh lemon juice
1 teaspoon onion powder
1 teaspoon salt (optional)

6 cups chopped broccoli

Place the potato in a saucepan with 1 cup of the water. Bring to a boil and cook until tender, about 15 minutes. Pour into a blender or food processor and process until smooth. Add 1 more cup of the water and the remaining sauce ingredients, except for the last 2 cups of water. Blend until smooth. Pour into a saucepan and mix well with the remaining 2 cups of water.

Meanwhile, steam the broccoli until tender, about 10 minutes. Drain well.

Cook the sauce mixture over medium heat, stirring constantly until thickened, 5 to 6 minutes.

Place the drained broccoli in a bowl and pour the sauce over it, mixing gently.

Potato Curry

SERVINGS: 6

PREPARATION TIME: 30 MINUTES (NEED COOKED POTATOES)

COOKING TIME: 15 MINUTES

1 large onion, chopped
2 cloves garlic, minced
1 tablespoon grated fresh
ginger
1 cup water
1 teaspoon ground cumin
1 teaspoon ground
coriander
½ teaspoon ground
turmeric
½ teaspoon Garam
Masala (page 277)

⅛ teaspoon cayenne
(optional)
4 cups chopped boiled
potatoes (4 to 5
potatoes)
2 cups frozen green peas,
thawed
2 to 3 tablespoons chopped
fresh cilantro
1 tablespoon fresh lemon
juice

Sauté the onion, garlic, and ginger in ½ cup of the water for 3 to 4 minutes, or until the onion softens slightly. Add the spices and cook, stirring, for 1 minute. Add the remaining ½ cup water, the potatoes, and the peas. Cook over low heat, uncovered, stirring frequently, for 10 minutes.

Remove from the heat and sprinkle with the cilantro and lemon juice before serving.

Thai Vegetable Curry

SERVINGS: 6 TO 8

PREPARATION TIME: 45 MINUTES   COOKING TIME: 20 MINUTES

Serve over brown rice. To be really authentic, coconut milk would be used in this recipe. Because of the high fat content of coconut milk, however, I have substituted soy milk. The vanilla-flavored ones work best tastewise.

1 stalk fresh lemon grass (see Note)

1 bay leaf

4 to 8 small red chili peppers (depending on how hot you like your curry)

⅓ cup water

2 tablespoons soy sauce

1⅔ cups vanilla-flavored soy milk

¼ pound green beans, cut into 1- to 2-inch pieces

2 small zucchini, cut in half lengthwise, then thickly sliced

2 small long eggplants, thickly sliced

½ pound broccoli, cut into florets

One 15-ounce can baby corn, drained

One 15-ounce can straw mushrooms, drained

1 tablespoon cornstarch, mixed with ¼ cup water

15 Thai basil leaves (see Note)

Grind the lemon grass, bay leaf, and chili peppers in a food processor or with a mortar and pestle. Place the ⅓ cup water and soy sauce in a large pot or wok. Add the pepper paste. Cook gently for 2 minutes. Add the soy milk and the fresh vegetables. Simmer, covered, for 15 minutes, stirring occasionally. Add the corn and mushrooms. Continue to cook for 2 minutes. Stir in the cornstarch mixture. Cook, stirring, until it thickens slightly. Stir in the whole basil leaves until they are slightly wilted.

Note: Lemon grass is a spice that grows in long stalks about ¼- to ½-inch thick and looks rather like a weed. Thai basil is usually more purple in color and has smaller leaves than common basil. Both can be found in Asian markets. If you cannot find these ingredients, use about 1 teaspoon freshly grated lemon zest in place of the lemon grass, and use slightly less common basil in place of the Thai (cut the leaves in half).

Cauliflower-Potato Curry

SERVINGS: 6 TO 8
PREPARATION TIME: 25 MINUTES
COOKING TIME: 1¼ HOURS

Serve over brown rice or other whole grains.

1 large onion, chopped
2 cloves garlic, minced
¼ cup water
1 tablespoon ground cumin
1 tablespoon chili powder
2 teaspoons curry powder
4 cups vegetable broth (page 132)
1 cup lentils

One 15-ounce can stewed tomatoes
2 medium potatoes, peeled and chopped
2 cups cauliflower florets
1 carrot, scrubbed and sliced
1 cup frozen green peas, thawed
¼ cup chopped fresh cilantro

Place the onion and garlic in a large pot with the water. Cook, stirring, for a couple of minutes, then add the spices and stir to coat. Add the vegetable stock and lentils. Mix well, bring to a boil, reduce the heat, cover, and cook for 30 minutes.

Add the tomatoes, potatoes, cauliflower, and carrot. Continue to cook for another 30 minutes. Stir in the peas. Cook for 5 minutes. Remove from the heat and stir in the cilantro.

Mu Shu Vegetables

SERVINGS: 8 TO 10

PREPARATION TIME: 20 MINUTES   COOKING TIME: 12 MINUTES

2 cups water
1 ounce dried shiitake mushrooms
6 leaves Chinese cabbage, thinly sliced
1 bunch baby bok choy or 3 leaves regular bok choy, thinly sliced
1 carrot, scrubbed and grated
4 scallions, thinly sliced lengthwise in 2-inch strips
1 cup mung bean sprouts

1 tablespoon grated fresh ginger
¼ cup soy sauce
2 tablespoons plum sauce
½ pound firm tofu, cut into thin strips
2 tablespoons cornstarch mixed with ¼ cup cold water
8 to 10 rice-paper disks (see Note), soaked in warm water for 5 minutes and drained between paper towels

Bring the water to a boil, pour over the mushrooms in a bowl, and let soak for 15 minutes, while you prepare the other vegetables. Drain the mushrooms, reserving the water. Cut off any hard stems and discard. Slice the mushrooms into thin strips.

Place ½ cup of the reserved mushroom liquid in a large pot or wok. Add the vegetables and ginger. Cook, stirring, for 5 minutes. Add the mushrooms, soy sauce, and plum sauce. Cook, stirring, for another 5 minutes. Add the tofu strips and cornstarch mixture. Cook, stirring, until thickened.

To serve, place a line of the vegetable mixture down the center of a rice-paper disk. Roll up and place, seam-side down, on a plate. Place a little plum sauce over the top, if desired, and eat with a fork.

Note: If you cannot find rice-paper disks (usually available in Oriental markets), use flour tortillas or wonton wrappers instead, provided they don't have eggs. Handle the rice-paper disks with care after soaking and draining. They tear easily.

Green Pepper and Tomato Teriyaki

SERVINGS: 6 TO 8
PREPARATION TIME: 30 MINUTES
COOKING TIME: 20 TO 25 MINUTES

Serve over brown rice or other whole grains.

1¾ cups water
1½ cups chopped onion
2 cloves garlic, minced
1½ cups quartered
   mushrooms
1 cup sliced celery
¼ cup unsweetened
   pineapple juice
¼ cup soy sauce

¼ cup cornstarch
1½ teaspoons honey
½ teaspoon grated fresh
   ginger
⅛ teaspoon crushed red
   pepper flakes
1½ cups green bell pepper
   strips
2 cups tomato wedges

Place ¾ cup of the water in a large pot. Add the onion and garlic and cook, stirring frequently, for 5 minutes. Add the mushrooms and celery. Cook, stirring, for 10 minutes. Mix the remaining 1 cup water with the pineapple juice, soy sauce, cornstarch, honey, ginger, and red pepper. Add to the sautéed vegetables. Cook, stirring, until thickened.

Add the green-pepper strips and tomato wedges. Cook over low heat for 5 minutes, stirring occasionally.

Harvest Vegetable Sauté

SERVINGS: 4
PREPARATION TIME: 25 MINUTES
COOKING TIME: 10 MINUTES

Serve over brown rice.

¼ cup water
2 tablespoons soy sauce
2 cloves garlic, pressed
1 teaspoon grated fresh ginger
Dash sesame oil
1 small onion, coarsely chopped
¼ pound mushrooms, sliced
1 cup small broccoli florets

1 cup small cauliflower florets
1 small yellow crookneck squash, cut in half and sliced
2 small zucchini, sliced
Additional ¾ cup water or broth to keep vegetables moist
Freshly ground pepper to taste

Heat the ¼ cup of water, soy sauce, garlic, ginger, and sesame oil to boiling in a wok or large pan. Add the onion and cook, stirring, until softened, about 2 minutes.

Add the remaining vegetables. Cook, stirring, until the vegetables are coated with sauce. Add the additional water and steam for 5 minutes, covered. Remove the cover and cook, stirring, for 2 minutes longer until all of the liquid is absorbed. Season to taste with pepper.

Vegetables Provençale

SERVINGS: 6
PREPARATION TIME: 25 MINUTES
COOKING TIME: 15 TO 20 MINUTES

2 small zucchini
2 ripe tomatoes
2 small thin or ½ large round eggplant
1 medium green bell pepper
1 small red onion
¼ pound mushrooms
⅓ cup water
1 clove garlic, minced
1 tablespoon tomato paste

Freshly ground pepper to taste
¼ cup chopped fresh parsley
¼ cup chopped fresh basil
1 teaspoon minced fresh thyme
½ teaspoon minced fresh rosemary
Balsamic vinegar (optional)

Wash and trim all of the vegetables and cut into ½-inch cubes. Place the ⅓ cup of water in a large heavy pot. Add the garlic and tomato paste. Heat, stirring, until well mixed. Add all of the vegetables. Cover and cook over low heat until the vegetables are tender but not mushy, about 15 minutes. Season with plenty of freshly ground pepper.

Combine the parsley, basil, thyme, and rosemary. Stir into the vegetables. Serve warm or cold, splashing on some balsamic vinegar just before serving, if desired.

Vegetable Quiche

SERVINGS: MAKES ONE 8-INCH PIE
PREPARATION TIME: 25 MINUTES
COOKING TIME: 45 MINUTES

1 onion, finely chopped
1 small green bell pepper, finely chopped
2 small carrots, scrubbed and finely chopped
Two 10-ounce packages firm tofu
1 tablespoon Worcestershire sauce
1 tablespoon soy sauce
2 teaspoons honey
1 teaspoon prepared mustard
1 teaspoon Mrs. Dash
2 ounces soy cheddar cheese, grated
1 zucchini, finely chopped
½ cup frozen green peas

Preheat the oven to 350°F.

Place the onion, green pepper, and carrot in a large bowl. Place one package of the tofu in a food processor or blender and add all of the seasonings and 1 ounce of the cheese. Process until smooth. Add to the vegetable mixture in the bowl and mix well.

Mash the second package of tofu with a potato masher and add to the vegetable mixture. Then add the zucchini and peas. Mix gently.

Pour into a nonstick 8-inch pie plate. Sprinkle the top with the remaining 1 ounce of soy cheese. Bake for 45 minutes, or until firmly set. Let cool 5 minutes before serving.

Pizza

MAKES ONE 16-INCH PIZZA (4 CUPS SAUCE)
PREPARATION TIME: 2 HOURS (TO MAKE CRUST AND SAUCE)
COOKING TIME: 20 TO 30 MINUTES

CRUST

1 cup warm water
1 package active dry
  yeast
1½ cups whole-wheat flour

1½ cups unbleached white
  flour
½ teaspoon salt
Cornmeal

SAUCE

4 cups crushed or strained
  tomatoes
1 teaspoon dried
  oregano

1 teaspoon dried basil, or
2 teaspoons chopped fresh
  basil
1 clove garlic, crushed

TOPPINGS

Sliced fresh mushrooms
Chopped green bell
  pepper
Chopped onion

Sliced water-packed
  artichoke hearts
Sliced zucchini
Chopped fresh spinach

Mix the yeast in the warm water. Stir and set aside for 5 to 10 minutes.

Put the flours and salt in a large mixing bowl. Stir to combine. Add the yeast mixture. Stir until the dough comes away from the sides of the bowl. Knead the dough in the bowl about 50 times. Turn the dough out of the bowl onto a well-floured board. Flour your hands well. Knead the dough until it is soft and springy and does not stick to your hands. Add more flour as necessary. Return the dough to the bowl. Cover with a damp towel and set in a warm place. Let rise for about 1 hour, or until doubled.

Remove the dough from the bowl and knead for a couple of minutes. Lightly oil the bottom of a 16-inch pizza pan or use a non-stick pan. Stretch the dough out until it is about half the size of the pan. Sprinkle the pan with cornmeal. Place the dough in the pan; spread and pat it out with your fingers and the heels of your hands. (If the dough is well floured, you can use a rolling pin.) Spread to the edge of the pan. Pull up enough so that a border is formed to keep the sauce in.

Preheat the oven to 400°F.

Combine all of the sauce ingredients in a bowl. Spread the sauce on the crust. Layer on the toppings of your choice. Bake for 20 minutes, or until the crust is brown.

Stuffed Pizza: Make a double recipe of pizza crust, and use a 13- or 14-inch deep-dish pizza pan. Roll out half of the dough until it is larger than the bottom of the deep-dish pan. Lightly oil the bottom of the pan and sprinkle with cornmeal. Place the dough in the pan, push it into the corners of the bottom, and let it overlap the sides.

Cover the dough with the toppings of your choice.

Roll out the other half of the dough just until it is large enough to cover the vegetable mixture. Take the bottom crust and overlap over the top crust. Pinch the edges together to make a border for the sauce. Cut a 1-inch slit in the top to allow steam to escape. Spread 1 cup of the sauce over the top crust. Bake at 400°F for 30 minutes, or until the crust is brown.

Macaroni and Cabbage

SERVINGS: 6
PREPARATION TIME: 40 MINUTES
COOKING TIME: 45 MINUTES

12 ounces whole-wheat
macaroni
5 quarts boiling water
1 medium onion,
chopped
1 cup water

1 small head cabbage,
coarsely chopped
One 28-ounce can whole
tomatoes
One 8-ounce can tomato
sauce

Preheat the oven to 350°F.

Drop the macaroni into the boiling water and cook until just tender, 8 to 10 minutes. Sauté the chopped onion in the 1 cup of water until transparent, about 5 minutes. Add the chopped cabbage and sauté until the cabbage is limp.

Lightly oil a casserole dish. Spread a layer of cooked macaroni on the bottom, followed by a layer of cabbage and onion. Repeat until all is used. Slightly chop the tomatoes while still in the can, then pour over the macaroni-cabbage mixture. Pour the tomato sauce over everything. Cover and bake for 45 minutes, or until the sauce appears to have thickened slightly.

Carrot Loaf or Crispy Carrot Burgers

SERVINGS: 6 TO 8

PREPARATION TIME: 45 MINUTES (NEED COOKED RICE AND BEANS)

COOKING TIME: 1 HOUR

Save this for special occasions—it's rich because of the high-fat tahini and soy milk. Top the loaf with marinara, mushroom gravy, or any other of your favorite sauces.

3 cups grated carrot

2 cups cooked brown rice

2 cups mashed cooked garbanzo beans

1 cup whole-wheat bread crumbs

⅓ cup tahini

1 cup finely chopped onion

1 cup finely chopped celery

½ cup finely chopped fresh parsley

1 tablespoon soy sauce

¼ cup vegetable broth or water

2 cloves garlic

4 teaspoons Ener-G Egg Replacer, well beaten with 8 tablespoons water

¼ cup soy milk

Preheat the oven to 350°F.

In a large bowl, mix the carrot, rice, garbanzo beans, bread crumbs, and tahini. In a saucepan, sauté the onion, celery, parsley, and soy sauce in the ¼ cup of stock or water for 5 minutes.

In a blender, puree the garlic cloves with the Egg Replacer/ water mixture.

Add all of the ingredients, including the soy milk, to the carrot mixture and mix well.

Press into a nonstick loaf pan and bake, uncovered, for 1 hour, or until it is firm to the touch. When cooked, put an oblong plate on top of the loaf pan and (using pot holders) hold the two together and turn them over quickly, allowing the loaf to drop out onto the plate.

To bake burger patties, form the mixture into 2-inch balls and flatten them onto a nonstick cookie sheet. Bake for 25 minutes, or until golden brown. Turn over and bake 10 to 15 minutes more, or until crispy brown.

Tzimmes

SERVINGS: 6 TO 8
PREPARATION TIME: 25 MINUTES
COOKING TIME: 55 MINUTES

I fell in love with this traditional Jewish holiday dish when it was served at a large holiday dinner at our church many years ago.

1 pound carrots, scrubbed and sliced 1 inch thick

6 medium yams, peeled and coarsely chopped

¾ cup pitted prunes or dried unsulphured apricots, or a combination of the two

1 cup fresh-squeezed orange juice

½ cup honey

½ teaspoon ground cinnamon

Preheat the oven to 350°F.

Place the carrots and yams in a large pot and add water to cover. Cook over medium heat for about 15 minutes, or until tender but still firm. Remove from the heat and drain.

Place the vegetables in a covered casserole dish. Add the prunes or apricots and mix gently.

Combine the orange juice, honey, and cinnamon. Pour over the vegetables and fruit. Cover and bake for 30 minutes. Uncover, stir gently, and continue to bake, uncovered, for another 10 minutes.

Spaghetti Squash Marinara

SERVINGS: 6
PREPARATION TIME: 30 MINUTES (NEED COOKED BEANS)
COOKING TIME: 45 MINUTES

½ cup water
1 onion, sliced
½ cup finely diced carrot
½ cup finely diced celery
2 tablespoons chili powder
2 tablespoons dried basil
1 tablespoon paprika
1 tablespoon minced fresh garlic

½ teaspoon ground nutmeg
One 16-ounce can stewed tomatoes
1½ cups cooked pinto beans or pink beans
1 medium bunch Swiss chard, stems removed, leaves coarsely chopped
1 large spaghetti squash

Place the water in a large pot or wok. Add the onion, carrot, celery, and the seasonings. Cook, stirring, over medium-high heat until the vegetables have softened slightly. Add the tomatoes and beans. Reduce the heat and cook over medium-low heat for 30 minutes. Add the Swiss chard and cook for an additional 10 minutes.

While the sauce is cooking, cut the squash in half, remove the seeds, and cook by one of the following methods:

1. Place in a large pot with 2 to 3 inches of water covering the bottom. Cover the pot and steam over medium heat for 30 minutes.
2. Place cut-side down in a baking dish and bake at 350°F for 45 minutes.
3. Microwave for 10 to 15 minutes at high power, cut-side up, in a dish with a small amount of water covering the bottom.

Pull out the cooked strands of the squash with a fork and arrange on a serving platter. Ladle the sauce over the spaghetti-squash strands.

Stuffed Winter Squash

SERVINGS: 4

PREPARATION TIME: 40 MINUTES (NEED COOKED BEANS)
COOKING TIME: 1 HOUR, 5 MINUTES

2 cups apricot nectar
½ teaspoon ground ginger
⅛ teaspoon ground coriander

4 servings winter squash (see Note)

STUFFING

1 cup sliced mushrooms
1 onion, chopped
1½ cups chopped celery
2 small apples, peeled and diced
1 cup apricot nectar
1 cup cooked white beans
2 tablespoons chopped fresh parsley

2 cloves garlic, pressed
1 tablespoon soy sauce
½ teaspoon Parsley Patch seasoning, general blend
½ teaspoon dried sage
⅛ teaspoon cayenne
2 to 3 cups whole-wheat bread cubes

Preheat the oven to 350°F.

In a bowl, stir together the 2 cups of nectar, ginger, and coriander. Set aside. Prepare the squash by cleaning and cutting into halves or pieces, depending on the kind used. Place in a large baking dish. Pour the apricot marinade over the squash. Bake, basting with marinade every 15 minutes, until easily pierced with a fork, about 45 minutes. Remove from the oven and keep warm by covering. Reduce the oven temperature to 300°F.

To prepare the stuffing: Sauté the mushrooms, onion, celery and apple in the apricot nectar for 10 minutes. Add the beans and all of the seasonings and simmer for a few minutes to allow the flavors to blend. Stir in the bread cubes. Transfer to a covered casserole dish and bake for 20 minutes.

Place the squash on a plate and serve with a scoop of stuffing.

Note: Use any of the following: 2 medium acorn squash, cut in half; 1 butternut squash, cut in half lengthwise then cut crosswise; or 1 large piece of banana squash or Hubbard squash, cut into 4 pieces.

Stuffed Cabbage Rolls

SERVINGS: 10 TO 12

PREPARATION TIME: 1 HOUR (NEED COOKED RICE)

COOKING TIME: 1½ HOURS

1 head cabbage
5 to 6 cups cooked brown rice
10 to 15 mushrooms, sliced
⅓ cup unsweetened pineapple juice
1 large onion, minced

4 cloves garlic, minced
⅓ cup water
¾ teaspoon dry mustard
¾ teaspoon caraway seeds
½ teaspoon dried sage

SAUCE

One 8-ounce can tomato sauce
5 tablespoons catsup
One 8-ounce can pineapple chunks, in their own juice
2 to 3 carrots, scrubbed and chopped
1 large apple, coarsely chopped
5 to 6 prunes, coarsely chopped

2 tablespoons brown-rice syrup
2 peaches, coarsely chopped
2 to 3 tablespoons fresh lemon juice
2 tablespoons brown sugar
4 teaspoons vegetable seasoning mix (e.g., Bernard Jensen's)
¾ cup water

Place the cabbage in a large pot with water to cover. Bring to a boil and cook for 5 minutes, or until the leaves peel off easily. Set aside. Combine the rice with the mushrooms and sauté for 3 to 4 minutes in the ⅓ cup pineapple juice. In a separate pan, sauté the onion and garlic in the ⅓ cup water for several minutes; add the seasonings. Mix well and add to the rice-mushroom mixture. Meanwhile, combine all of the ingredients for the sauce in a medium saucepan. Bring to a boil, then remove from the heat and set aside.

Peel off cabbage leaves one by one and place a small amount of the rice mixture in each leaf (from 1 to 2 tablespoons, depending on the size of the leaf). Fold the sides over, roll up, and secure with a toothpick. Place the rolls in the bottom of a large pot. Pour the sauce over the rolls and top with cabbage leaves too small to stuff. Simmer over low heat for about 1½ hours, or until tender.

Tempeh-Stuffed Peppers

SERVINGS: 4

PREPARATION TIME: 20 MINUTES (NEED COOKED RICE)

COOKING TIME: 45 MINUTES

4 green or red bell peppers, cleaned, tops removed

One 8-ounce package tempeh, either plain or with quinoa, crumbled

One 8- to 10-ounce jar salsa

1 cup cooked brown rice

One 4-ounce can chopped green chilies

2 ounces soy cheddar cheese, grated

Preheat the oven to 350°F.

Mix the tempeh with half of the salsa, the rice, chilies, and half of the cheese. Stuff this mixture into the bell peppers. Pour the remaining salsa over the peppers and sprinkle with the remaining cheese.

Place the peppers in a casserole dish and bake until they are cooked and tender, about 45 minutes.

Zucchini and Eggplant–Stuffed Tomatoes

SERVINGS: 8
PREPARATION TIME: 45 MINUTES
COOKING TIME: 30 MINUTES

8 ripe tomatoes
⅓ cup water
1 tablespoon soy sauce
½ cup chopped onion
2 cloves garlic, minced
1 cup chopped yellow crookneck squash
2 cups chopped zucchini
¾ cup chopped eggplant

1 cup reserved chopped tomato "meat"
2 tablespoons minced fresh basil
Freshly ground pepper to taste
1 tablespoon minced fresh parsley

Preheat the oven to 350°F.

Cut the tops off the tomatoes and scoop out the insides, reserving the tomato "meat." (Place in a strainer to drain off as much of the liquid as possible.) Set the tomatoes aside.

Place the water in a saucepan. Add the soy sauce, bring to a boil, and add the onion and garlic. Cook, stirring, for 2 minutes, then add the squash, zucchini, and eggplant. Cook for another 5 minutes, then add the remaining ingredients. Cook for another 2 minutes and remove from the heat.

Stuff the mixture into the tomatoes. Top with the bread-crumb mixture of your choice (page 128). Place in a baking dish with a small amount of water covering the bottom. Bake for 20 minutes, or until the tomatoes pierce easily with a fork.

Note: These may be "held" in a low-temperature oven for an hour or so after the initial baking time. They also reheat well a day or two later. Reheat in a microwave, covered with plastic wrap, until heated through, about 3 minutes on high, or reheat in a steamer basket over boiling water for about 5 minutes.

Stuffed Collard Greens

SERVINGS: 6 TO 8

PREPARATION TIME: 45 MINUTES, PLUS OVERNIGHT SOAKING

COOKING TIME: 1½ HOURS

1 bunch large collard
leaves

FILLING

½ cup adzuki beans (see
Note 1)
1½ cups water
1 cup short-grain brown
rice
2 cups vegetable stock or
water

1 medium onion, minced
½ cup shredded carrot
1 to 2 tablespoons minced
fresh ginger

SAUCE

6 large tomatoes, pureed
in a blender
1 small onion, chopped
2 cloves garlic, crushed

1 tablespoon fresh basil
or oregano
One 1-inch cinnamon stick
3 whole cloves

Soak the beans overnight in water to cover. Drain. Place in a medium saucepan with the 1½ cups of water. Bring to a boil, cover, reduce the heat, and cook for 1 hour. Meanwhile, bring the stock or water to a boil. Add the rice, reduce the heat, and cook, covered, for 1 hour.

Lightly wash the collard greens. Steam for 1 minute to soften slightly. Cut off the center stems and cut each leaf into two or three good-sized pieces. Set aside.

Combine the sauce ingredients in a large covered saucepan. Set aside.

Drain the beans, mash with a potato masher, and place in a large bowl. Add the cooked rice and mix well. Add the remaining filling ingredients and mix. Place 2 to 3 tablespoons of filling on each collard piece and roll up into neat bundles. Place the bundles in the pan with the sauce. Bring to a gentle boil, reduce the heat, cover, and simmer for 30 minutes, spooning sauce over the rolls occasionally.

Discard the cloves and cinnamon stick before serving. To serve, place the collard rolls on a plate and spoon a little sauce over each roll.

Note: 1. Adzuki beans are small dark red beans, more common in Asia. If your local natural-food store doesn't have them, look for them in an Asian market.

2. If there is any leftover filling, it may be frozen for later use, added to soups or stews, or used as a base for sauces or gravies.

Peperonata

SERVINGS: 8 TO 10 (2 QUARTS)
PREPARATION TIME: 25 MINUTES
COOKING TIME: 15 TO 18 MINUTES

Serve over pasta.

4 medium onions, cut in half lengthwise, then sliced into thin strips
4 to 5 cloves garlic, sliced
¼ teaspoon crushed red pepper flakes
2 cups vegetable broth (page 132) or water
6 yellow, red, and green bell peppers, cut into strips
4 bay leaves

2 tablespoons light barley miso
4 tomatoes, peeled and chopped, or one 28-ounce can whole tomatoes, chopped
1 tablespoon arrowroot, dissolved in ¼ cup water
Freshly ground black pepper to taste

Sauté the onions, garlic, and crushed pepper in ½ cup of the stock for 5 minutes. Add the pepper strips, bay leaves, and ½ cup more stock, and cook for 5 minutes over medium heat, stirring often.

Dissolve the miso in ½ cup stock. Add to the vegetable mixture, along with the chopped tomatoes and the remaining ½ cup stock, and cook for 5 to 7 minutes longer. Push the peppers aside; add the dissolved arrowroot mixture to the liquid and stir to thicken. Add black pepper to taste.

Layered Vegetable Casserole

SERVINGS: 6 TO 8
PREPARATION TIME: 40 MINUTES
COOKING TIME: 1 HOUR

4 large potatoes (russets or
  yellow Finns, which are
  lovely and sweet)
2 large sweet potatoes
1 large butternut squash

4 medium zucchini
2 medium red onions
A few sprinkles dried dill
or a sprig or two fresh dill
(optional)

Preheat the oven to 350°F.

Scrub the potatoes and cut them into ¼-inch slices. Peel the sweet potatoes and cut them into ¼-inch slices. Peel the squash and cut it into ¼-inch slices. Trim the ends of the zucchini and cut them into ¼-inch slices. Peel and thinly slice the red onions and separate the rings.

Pour a thin layer of water in the bottom of a large casserole dish. Layer half the vegetables in the order given, and top with a sprinkle of dill. Repeat with another layer of each. Cover and bake for 1 hour, or until vegetables pierce easily with a fork.

Variation: 2 cups of sliced carrots are a good addition or a replacement for either the squash or sweet potatoes.

Spanish-Style Vegetable Casserole

SERVINGS: 4
PREPARATION TIME: 20 MINUTES
COOKING TIME: 50 MINUTES

The woman who sent me this recipe tells me that it's always a big hit when she makes it for her family. Feel free to substitute other vegetables for the ones listed below. John suggests that a few cubes of pineapple would make an interesting addition. A few sprinkles of soy sauce over the top may be used for extra seasoning.

1 to 2 tablespoons water
1 medium onion, chopped
1 clove garlic, minced
1 medium tomato, cored and chopped
1 medium red or green bell pepper, chopped
1 potato, peeled and diced
½ teaspoon paprika
⅛ to ¼ teaspoon cayenne
1 cup long-grain brown rice
2 cups vegetable broth or water
2 medium carrots, scrubbed and chopped or sliced
1 to 2 zucchini, chopped
2 cups frozen green peas

Heat the water in a large heavy saucepan. Add the onion and garlic and cook for 1 minute. Mix in the tomato and pepper and cook for about 3 minutes. Add the potato, paprika, and cayenne (use less if you don't like spicy foods) and cook for 2 minutes longer. Stir in the rice, vegetable broth, and carrot and adjust the heat so the mixture bubbles gently. Cover and simmer for 15 minutes. Stir in the zucchini and peas. Cover and cook for another 30 minutes.

Garden Pitas

SERVINGS: 4 LARGE
PREPARATION TIME: 30 MINUTES
COOKING TIME: 30 MINUTES

Serve hot, topped with a warm sauce, such as Szechwan Sauce or a mush-room sauce, or an oil-free dressing.

½ cup water
1 tablespoon soy sauce
1 small onion, chopped
1 teaspoon finely chopped fresh basil
2 cups chopped broccoli

2 cups packed washed spinach leaves
½ pound mushrooms, sliced
2 medium tomatoes, sliced
4 whole-wheat pita breads

Place the water, soy sauce, onion, and basil in a frying pan. Cook, stirring, over medium heat for 2 to 3 minutes, or until the onion softens slightly. Add the broccoli and continue to cook, stirring, for another 6 to 8 minutes, until the broccoli is tender-crisp. Remove from the heat.

Preheat the oven to 350°F.

Place the pita breads on a baking sheet, rounded side down, so a small bowl is formed. Divide the broccoli-onion mixture among the four pitas. Lay the spinach leaves over the broccoli mixture; then layer the sliced mushrooms over the spinach, finishing with the sliced tomatoes.

Bake for 30 minutes, or until the vegetables pierce easily with a fork.

Potato Burritos

SERVINGS: 6 TO 8
PREPARATION TIME: 30 MINUTES
COOKING TIME: 30 MINUTES

6 cups Chunky
Enchilada Sauce (page
336)
12 whole-wheat tortillas
or 12 to 14 soft corn
tortillas
3 cups mashed potatoes
(recipe follows)

1 cup chopped scallion
1 cup frozen corn
kernels, thawed
One 4-ounce can chopped
green chilies

Preheat the oven to 350°F.

Spread 1 cup of the sauce over the bottom of a casserole dish. Spread a line of potatoes down the center of each tortilla. Sprinkle on some scallion, corn, and green chilies. Roll up and place, seam-side down, in the casserole. Repeat until all of the ingredients are used. Pour the remaining sauce over the tortillas. Cover and bake for 30 minutes, or until the sauce is bubbly.

MASHED POTATOES

SERVINGS: MAKES 3 CUPS

12 medium potatoes,
peeled

¼ to ½ cup salsa (optional)

Chop the potatoes coarsely and place them in a saucepan with water to cover. Cook until the potatoes are tender, 20 to 30 minutes. Drain off the water, reserving 2 cups. Mash the potatoes with a small amount of the water until they are creamy. Stir in some salsa, if desired, for a more Mexican flavor.

Tex-Mex Vegetable Burritos

SERVINGS: 4
PREPARATION TIME: 15 MINUTES
COOKING TIME: 10 MINUTES

1 bunch scallions, cut into
1-inch pieces
1 green bell pepper, sliced
into strips
1 red bell pepper, sliced into
strips
½ cup water
1 cup frozen corn kernels,
thawed

2 teaspoons cornstarch
1 cup salsa
12 cherry tomatoes, cut in
half
4 large whole-wheat tortillas
Fresh cilantro sprigs
(optional)

Sauté the scallions and the peppers in the water for 2 minutes. Add the corn and cook for another 2 to 3 minutes.

Mix the cornstarch into the salsa and add to the vegetables. Cook, stirring, until thickened. Add the tomatoes and cook for 1 minute longer.

To serve, place a line of the vegetable mixture down the center of a tortilla, and top with sprigs of cilantro, if desired. Roll up and eat.

Burritos de Legumbres

SERVINGS: 4
PREPARATION TIME: 15 MINUTES
COOKING TIME: 10 MINUTES

This was inspired by a wonderful vegetable burrito that I often order at a Mexican restaurant in North Lake Tahoe.

1 bunch scallions, cut into ½-inch pieces

2 zucchini, cut in half, then sliced ½ inch thick

¼ pound mushrooms, sliced

1 cup small broccoli florets

1 leek, washed and sliced, or 1 small onion, coarsely chopped

¾ cup water

⅛ cup packed chopped fresh cilantro (optional)

One 7-ounce can Mexican green sauce

1 tablespoon cornstarch, mixed with 2 tablespoons water

8 whole-wheat flour tortillas

Fresh Salsa (page 339) (optional)

Sauté all of the vegetables in ½ cup of the water for 5 minutes, until tender-crisp. Add the cilantro, green sauce, and the remaining ¼ cup water, and mix well. Add the cornstarch mixture. Cook, stirring, until thickened.

Place a line of the vegetable mixture down the center of a tortilla. Add a spoonful of salsa, if desired. Roll up and eat.

Main Dish Pastas

Teriyaki Pasta

SERVINGS: 6 TO 8
PREPARATION TIME: 20 MINUTES
COOKING TIME: 12 TO 15 MINUTES

½ pound whole-wheat
    spaghetti
5 cups boiling water
3 medium carrots, scrubbed

3 medium zucchini
½ pound mushrooms, sliced
½ cup teriyaki sauce

Drop the spaghetti into the boiling water and cook, uncovered, for 10 minutes.

Cut the carrots and zucchini into long, thin julienne strips to resemble spaghetti. After the spaghetti has cooked for 10 minutes, drop the vegetables into the water with the spaghetti. Cook for an additional 2 to 5 minutes. (Test the spaghetti during this time to see if it is done). Drain. Pour the teriyaki sauce over the pasta and vegetables, and toss to mix. Serve at once.

Oriental Pasta

SERVINGS: 4
PREPARATION TIME: 20 MINUTES
COOKING TIME: 20 MINUTES

1 to 2 cloves garlic, crushed
1 teaspoon grated fresh ginger
⅛ to ¼ teaspoon crushed red pepper flakes
2 carrots, scrubbed and sliced
1 medium bunch broccoli, cut into florets

½ cup water
¼ cup soy sauce
½ pound mushrooms, quartered
1 bunch scallions, cut into 1-inch pieces
½ pound soba noodles
1 tablespoon cornstarch, mixed with 2 tablespoons cold water

Place the garlic, ginger, red pepper, carrots, and broccoli in a wok or large pan with the ½ cup water and 2 tablespoons of the soy sauce. Cook, stirring, for 5 minutes. Add the mushrooms and scallions. Cook, covered, for about 10 minutes.

Prepare the pasta according to the package directions. Drain. Toss with the remaining 2 tablespoons of soy sauce.

Add the cornstarch mixture to the vegetable mixture. Cook, stirring, until thickened. Add to the pasta. Mix well.

Pasta Primavera

SERVINGS: 6
PREPARATION TIME: 30 MINUTES
COOKING TIME: 45 MINUTES

SAUCE

½ cup water
1 onion, chopped
2 stalks celery, chopped
2 cloves garlic, crushed
One 28-ounce can whole tomatoes, chopped, with liquid
1 tablespoon chopped fresh basil
1 tablespoon chopped fresh oregano
¼ cup chopped fresh parsley
One 8-ounce can tomato sauce

VEGETABLES

½ cup water
1 cup broccoli florets
1 cup asparagus or green beans, cut into 1-inch pieces
1 cup sliced zucchini or yellow squash
2 cups sliced mushrooms
Freshly ground black pepper
1 tablespoon soy sauce
1 pound uncooked whole-wheat or spinach pasta
2 quarts water

To make the sauce: Place the water in a medium saucepan. Add the onion, celery, and garlic. Cook over medium heat for 6 minutes, stirring often. Add the remaining ingredients. Reduce the heat and simmer for 30 minutes.

While the sauce cooks, put the water for the pasta on to boil and begin to cook the vegetables.

To cook the vegetables: Place the water in a nonstick wok or frying pan. Bring to a boil and add the broccoli and asparagus. Stir, cover, and steam for 4 minutes, or until softened slightly. Add the zucchini, mushrooms, pepper, and soy sauce. Stir and cook, uncovered, for an additional 4 minutes. Remove from the heat.

To cook the pasta: Bring the water to a boil in a large pot. Drop the pasta into the water. Stir to make sure all of the strands are separated. Cook until just tender, about 8 minutes. Drain.

To serve: Place the pasta on a plate. Layer on some of the vegetables and finish with a generous topping of the sauce.

Olivia's Vegetable Pasta

SERVINGS: 6 TO 8
PREPARATION TIME: 15 MINUTES (NEED COOKED POTATOES)
COOKING TIME: 15 MINUTES

The women who sent us this recipe say that this is one of their all-time favorite meals. They named it after the one who had the most input into creating it.

5 to 6 cloves garlic, finely chopped
Crushed red pepper flakes to taste
½ to ¾ cup finely chopped fresh basil
1 to 2 tablespoons soy sauce
6 quarts water

¾ pound vegetable fusille
4 cups rinsed and drained frozen mixed vegetables (no corn)
2 large red potatoes (scrubbed, cooked, and cubed; see Note)

Place the garlic, red pepper, basil, and soy sauce in a 1-quart saucepan. Set aside. In a 10-quart pot, bring the water to a boil and cook the pasta for 5 minutes. Add the mixed vegetables and cook for an additional 5 minutes.

Drain the pasta and vegetables, making sure to save a couple of cups of the cooking water. Add 1 cup of the cooking water to the garlic/basil mixture and heat it in the saucepan. Pour the heated mixture over the pasta and vegetables. Add the cooked potatoes. Mix all of the ingredients together, adding reserved cooking water as needed for moisture

Note: Cook the potatoes whole in a microwave oven on high for 6 minutes just before making this recipe. This tastes best if the potatoes are still warm when added to the pasta and vegetables.

Vegetable Lasagna

SERVINGS: 8 TO 10

PREPARATION TIME: 1½ HOURS   COOKING TIME: 1 HOUR

1 recipe Marinara Sauce (page 353)

4 cups fresh spinach (about 1 pound), or two 10-ounce packages frozen spinach

¼ teaspoon ground nutmeg

Three 10½-ounce packages firm tofu

2 tablespoons fresh lemon juice

1 teaspoon salt (optional)

¼ teaspoon freshly ground black pepper

1 tablespoon balsamic vinegar

1 teaspoon onion powder

6 quarts water

Two 10-ounce packages whole-wheat lasagna

3 medium to large zucchini (about 2 pounds)

3 teaspoons dried marjoram

3 teaspoons dried basil

3 teaspoons minced garlic

Begin by making the marinara sauce. While the sauce is simmering, wash and trim the fresh spinach, or defrost the frozen spinach. Chop and steam until barely tender, about 2 minutes. Drain well and toss while adding the nutmeg. Set aside.

Drain the tofu and crumble the contents of two of the boxes into a food processor or blender. Pulse only until the mixture is slightly lumpy. Crumble the remaining tofu into the mixture and add the salt, pepper, vinegar, and onion powder. Taste and adjust seasonings. Set aside.

Bring the water to a rapid boil. Add the lasagna separately to prevent the noodles from sticking together. Stir gently with a wooden spoon two or three times. Cook for 6 minutes, or until slightly undercooked. Drain, rinse under cold water, and lay out on damp towels. Cover with towels to prevent drying.

Wash and dry the zucchini and cut off the ends. Grate in a food processor or with a hand grater.

Preheat the oven to 350°F.

To assemble the lasagna, place a thin layer of sauce on the bottom of a 13 × 10-inch baking dish. Layer three or four noodles on top of the sauce. Cover with a thick masking of the tofu mixture. Top with a layer of zucchini, followed by a dotting of spinach and a sprinkling of marjoram, basil, and garlic granules. Repeat layers of tomato sauce, pasta, tofu mixture, zucchini, spinach, and seasonings twice more. End with a layer of pasta (three noodles), a layer of the tofu mixture, then a layer of marinara. Dust with herbs.

Cover with foil, lined with parchment paper, and bake for 45 minutes. Remove the cover and continue baking for 15 minutes, or until the sauce is bubbly. Cool 15 minutes before cutting.

Zucchini Lasagna

SERVINGS: 8
PREPARATION TIME: 40 MINUTES
COOKING TIME: 40 MINUTES

In this recipe, the zucchini takes the place of wheat noodles. This is a lighter version of traditional lasagna and is excellent for those who are allergic to wheat. (Replace bread crumbs with Wheat-Free Bread Crumbs, if desired.)

½ pound tofu, frozen and thawed (see Note, page 269)
2 tablespoons onion powder
¼ cup fresh lemon juice
1 cup diced onion
3 tablespoons minced garlic
2 tablespoons soy sauce
2 tablespoons chopped fresh basil

2 tablespoons Parsley Patch seasoning, general blend
1 bunch spinach, washed and trimmed
4 zucchini, sliced lengthwise ¼ inch thick
6 cups Marinara Sauce (page 353)
1½ cups seasoned bread crumbs (see page 128)

Preheat the oven to 350°F.

Press as much water out of the tofu as possible, then cut it into cubes. Sauté the tofu and onion powder in the lemon juice until lightly browned. Add the onion, garlic, soy sauce, basil, and Parsley Patch seasoning. Sauté for about 5 minutes longer. Stir in the spinach and sauté until limp, 1 to 2 minutes.

Place a small amount of the Marinara Sauce in the bottom of a 13 × 9-inch nonstick baking dish. Lay the zucchini over the sauce, followed by layers of the sautéed mixture, the sauce, the zucchini, and the sautéed mixture. Top with the rest of the Marinara Sauce and sprinkle with bread crumbs.

Bake for 40 minutes, or until lightly browned and bubbly.

Tricolor Lasagna

SERVINGS: 8 TO 10
PREPARATION TIME: 45 MINUTES
COOKING TIME: 30 MINUTES

3 quarts water
9 to 10 whole-wheat lasagna
noodles
2 tablespoons crushed
garlic
½ teaspoon dried
oregano
½ teaspoon dried basil
¼ teaspoon dried thyme

2 teaspoons parsley
flakes
4 cups tomato sauce
4 medium zucchini,
sliced in half
lengthwise
2 to 3 cups spinach, washed
3 cups Mockzarella
Cheese (page 124)

Preheat the oven to 400°F.

Bring the water to a boil. Add the lasagna noodles and cook until tender, about 8 minutes. Drain and set aside.

Mix the garlic and herbs into the tomato sauce and set aside.

Place 1 cup of the sauce in the bottom of a 13 × 9-inch baking dish. Arrange half of the zucchini over the sauce, then layer half of the spinach over the zucchini. Next layer half of the lasagna noodles over the vegetables. Spread half of the cheese over the lasagna noodles. Follow with another cup of the sauce, then repeat the zucchini, spinach, lasagna noodles, and cheese layers. Finish with the final 2 cups of the sauce.

Bake, uncovered, for 30 minutes, or until lightly browned and bubbly. Serve *immediately*.

Pasta Provençale

SERVINGS: 6
PREPARATION TIME: 8 TO 10 MINUTES
COOKING TIME: 12 TO 14 MINUTES

Two 15-ounce cans stewed
   tomatoes (see Note)
One 19-ounce can white
   beans or garbanzos,
   drained and rinsed

5 quarts water
One 10-ounce package
   spinach rotelle
¼ cup chopped fresh
   parsley

Place the tomatoes and beans in a saucepan and heat gently for 8 to 10 minutes.

Meanwhile, heat the water to boiling. Add the pasta and cook, uncovered, at a rapid boil for 12 to 14 minutes. Drain. Place in a large bowl. Add the tomato-bean sauce and toss to mix. Sprinkle with fresh parsley before serving.

Note: Try using Italian-, Mexican-, or Cajun-style stewed tomatoes.

Main Dish Grains

Savory Baked Polenta

SERVINGS: 6 TO 8
PREPARATION TIME: 5 MINUTES
COOKING TIME: 30 MINUTES
RESTING TIME: 30 MINUTES

Serve with Eggplant-Mushroom Sauce, Ratatouille, or another of your favorite sauces.

4 cups water	1 teaspoon chili powder
1 cup cornmeal	¼ teaspoon ground cumin
1 tablespoon soy sauce	

Preheat the oven to 400°F.

Place the water in a medium saucepan and bring to a boil. Reduce the heat to low and gradually stir in the cornmeal. Add the remaining ingredients and cook, stirring constantly, until very thick, about 10 minutes.

Pour into a nonstick 8 × 8-inch baking dish and flatten with a spatula. Bake for 20 minutes, or until set. Remove from the oven and let rest for 30 minutes. Remove from the pan and cut into squares. May be refrigerated at this point and reheated later.

To reheat, place in a microwave oven and heat for about 30 seconds on high power for each square. Or brown pieces on a nonstick griddle for about 5 minutes.

Broccoli-Barley Toss

SERVINGS: 8

PREPARATION TIME: 30 MINUTES

COOKING TIME: 1 HOUR

1 cup barley
3 cups vegetable broth (page 132) or water
2 cups broccoli florets
2 cups sliced mushrooms
1 cup snow peas, trimmed
½ cup sliced scallion
¼ cup chopped red bell pepper

¼ cup chopped green bell pepper
1 cup bean sprouts
¼ cup soy sauce
¼ cup water
¼ teaspoon ground ginger
1 tablespoon cornstarch, mixed with 2 tablespoons cold water

Place the barley and vegetable stock in a saucepan. Cover and cook over medium heat for 1 hour. About 15 minutes before the barley is done, place all of the vegetables, except the bean sprouts, in a large pot or wok with the soy sauce, water, and ginger. Cook, stirring, for 5 minutes. Add the bean sprouts and cook, stirring, for another 5 minutes. Add the cornstarch mixture and cook, stirring, until thickened, about 1 minute. Remove from the heat. Toss the vegetables with the cooked barley. Serve hot.

Mideast Pilaf Roll-Ups

SERVINGS: 6 TO 8
PREPARATION TIME: 30 MINUTES
COOKING TIME: 1½ HOURS

3 to 4 scallions, chopped
¼ cup water
3 cups vegetable broth
¾ cup long-grain brown rice
½ cup bulghur
14 to 16 romaine leaves or large spinach leaves

½ teaspoon ground cinnamon
⅓ cup currants
¼ cup pine nuts (optional)

Cook the scallions in the water in a medium saucepan until tender, 2 to 3 minutes. Add the broth, rice, and bulghur. Bring to a boil, reduce the heat, cover, and simmer for 45 to 50 minutes, or until tender. Remove from the heat and set aside for 10 minutes.

Steam the romaine leaves over boiling water for 2 minutes. Trim the stems. (Spinach leaves do not have to be steamed.)

Preheat the oven to 350°F.

Stir the cinnamon, currants, and pine nuts into the rice mixture.

Put a heaping tablespoon of the filling into each leaf or two, depending on the size of the leaf. Roll up tightly and place, seam-side down, in a baking dish. Add a small amount of broth or water to the bottom of the baking dish—just enough to cover the bottom. (This helps to keep the rolls moist.) Cover and bake for 30 minutes.

Spinach-Rice Enchiladas

SERVINGS: 6 TO 8
PREPARATION TIME: 30 MINUTES (NEED COOKED RICE)
COOKING TIME: 40 MINUTES

¼ cup water	1 tablespoon soy sauce
1 onion, chopped	1 teaspoon ground
2 cups chopped	cumin
washed spinach	5 to 6 cups Enchilada Sauce
3 cups cooked brown	(page 336)
rice	10 to 12 soft corn tortillas

Place the water and onion in a medium saucepan. Sauté until the onion softens slightly. Add the spinach. Cover and steam until just tender, 4 to 5 minutes. Remove from the heat. Add the rice and the seasonings. Mix and set aside.

Preheat the oven to 350°F.

Spread 1 cup of the sauce over the bottom of a casserole dish. Spread a line of the spinach-rice mixture down the center of a tortilla. Roll up and place, seam-side down, in the casserole. Repeat until all of the ingredients are used. Pour the remaining sauce over the tortillas. Cover and bake for 30 minutes.

Mexican Rice

SERVINGS: 6 TO 8
PREPARATION TIME: 15 MINUTES (NEED COOKED RICE)
COOKING TIME: 20 MINUTES

Serve plain or rolled up in a burrito shell, with salsa spooned over the top, if desired.

1 onion, chopped	1 bunch scallions,
1 green bell pepper,	chopped
chopped	

½ pound mushrooms,
sliced
2 cloves garlic, minced
½ cup water
One 16-ounce can chopped
tomatoes

One 4-ounce can chopped
green chilies
2 teaspoons chili powder
1 teaspoon ground cumin
Dash or two Tabasco
5 cups cooked brown rice

Sauté the onion, green pepper, scallion, mushrooms, and garlic in
the ½ cup of water for 10 minutes. Add the remaining ingredients
and mix well. Cook over low heat for about 10 minutes, or until
heated through, stirring frequently.

Vegetarian Paella

SERVINGS: 4
PREPARATION TIME: 15 MINUTES
COOKING TIME: 55 MINUTES

½ cup water
1 onion, coarsely chopped
8 medium mushrooms,
sliced
2 small zucchini, cut in half,
then sliced ½ inch thick
1 leek, washed and sliced
2 large cloves garlic,
crushed
1 medium tomato, coarsely
chopped

3 cups vegetable broth or
water
1¼ cups long-grain brown
rice
½ teaspoon crushed saffron
threads (or turmeric)
Generous grind of black
pepper
½ cup frozen green peas
Chopped fresh parsley for
garnish

Place the water in a large wok or Dutch oven. Add the onion and
sauté until most of the liquid is absorbed. Add the mushrooms,
zucchini, leek, and garlic. Stir constantly until the vegetables soften
slightly, 2 to 3 minutes. Add the tomato, broth, rice, saffron, and pepper. Bring to a boil, reduce the heat, and simmer, covered, for 30 minutes. Add the peas and continue to cook for another 5 to 10 minutes.
Turn off the heat and let rest for 10 minutes to allow any excess moisture to be absorbed. Sprinkle with parsley just before serving.

Wild Rice and Vegetable Pilaf

SERVINGS: 6
PREPARATION TIME: 20 MINUTES
COOKING TIME: 1 HOUR

½ cup water
1 to 2 cloves garlic, minced
1 cup chopped scallion
1 cup chopped cauliflower
1 cup chopped broccoli
1 potato, scrubbed and chopped
2 tablespoons soy sauce

1 cup long-grain brown rice
⅓ cup wild rice
3 cups vegetable broth
2 small zucchini, chopped
½ cup grated carrot
⅛ teaspoon sesame oil
¼ cup chopped fresh cilantro

Heat the water to boiling in a large saucepan. Add the garlic, scallion, cauliflower, broccoli, and potato. Cook, stirring, for 2 to 3 minutes. Add the soy sauce and cook for 1 minute longer. Add both kinds of rice and the vegetable broth. Bring to a boil, reduce the heat, cover, and cook for 15 minutes. Stir in the zucchini. After another 15 minutes, stir in the carrot. Continue to cook for 15 minutes. Stir in the sesame oil and cilantro. Mix and serve.

Bulghur-Stuffed Peppers

SERVINGS: 4
PREPARATION TIME: 30 MINUTES (NEED COOKED BEANS)
COOKING TIME: 30 MINUTES, PLUS 30 MINUTES RESTING TIME

4 green or red bell peppers
1 cup bulghur
1½ cups Light Vegetable Broth (page 133)
1 teaspoon minced fresh rosemary
1 teaspoon minced fresh thyme

1 teaspoon minced fresh marjoram
1 tomato, chopped
4 scallions, finely chopped
1 cup cooked beans (any kind)

Cut off the tops of the peppers and clean out the insides. Reserve the tops. Steam the peppers and tops over boiling water for 5 minutes. Remove from the heat and set aside.

Place the bulghur, broth, and fresh herbs in a medium saucepan. Bring to a boil, then turn off the heat, cover, and let rest for 30 minutes. Stir in the tomato, scallions, and cooked beans.

Preheat the oven to 350°F.

Fill the peppers with the bulghur mixture and replace the tops. Put about ½ inch of water or tomato juice in the bottom of a baking dish. Arrange the peppers in the dish; cover. Bake for 25 to 30 minutes, or until heated through.

Quick-Sautéed Spiced Vegetables with Rice

SERVINGS: 6
PREPARATION TIME: 20 MINUTES (NEED COOKED RICE)
COOKING TIME: 15 MINUTES

2 cloves garlic, crushed
2 teaspoons grated fresh ginger
½ cup water
1 carrot, scrubbed and sliced
¼ pound green beans, trimmed and cut into 1-inch pieces
½ pound mushrooms, sliced

2 zucchini, cut in half lengthwise and sliced
1 bunch scallions, cut into 1-inch pieces
4 cups cooked brown rice
3 tablespoons soy sauce
Dash sesame oil (optional)
Freshly ground pepper (optional)

Place the garlic and ginger in a large pot or wok with the water. Add the carrot and green beans. Sauté for 3 minutes. Add the mushrooms, and sauté for another 2 minutes. Add the zucchini and scallions. Stir, cover, reduce the heat, and cook until the vegetables are tender-crisp, 6 to 8 minutes, stirring frequently. Add the rice, soy sauce, and sesame oil, if desired. Mix well. Cook, stirring, over low heat until heated through. Sprinkle with pepper before serving, if desired.

Spanish Rice

SERVINGS: 4 TO 6
PREPARATION TIME: 10 MINUTES (NEED COOKED RICE)
COOKING TIME: 15 MINUTES

¼ cup water
1 onion, diced
1 green bell pepper, diced
3 cloves garlic, minced
One 15- to 16-ounce can
   whole tomatoes,
   chopped

1 tablespoon chili powder
2 teaspoons ground cumin
1 teaspoon dried basil
½ teaspoon Parsley Patch
   seasoning, general blend
¼ teaspoon cayenne
2 cups cooked brown rice

Place the water, onion, green pepper, and garlic in a medium sauce-pan. Cook, stirring, until softened, about 5 minutes. Add the toma-toes and seasonings. Cook for another 5 minutes. Add the cooked rice. Mix well. Heat for another 5 minutes to allow the flavors to blend.

Rice and Noodle Pilaf

SERVINGS: 6 TO 8
PREPARATION TIME: 5 MINUTES
COOKING TIME: 35 TO 45 MINUTES

In the Middle East, a pilaf or rice dish accompanies almost every meal. This type of dish is very often served at feasts. Serve with a bean-based soup, such as Curried Red Lentil Soup or Adas Bi Sabaanikh.

1 cup whole-wheat noodles
2 cups long-grain brown
   rice
6½ cups vegetable broth
   (page 132) or water

1 teaspoon ground cumin
½ teaspoon dried oregano

Break the noodles up into very small pieces, about ⅛ inch long. (Put them in a towel or bag and crush with a rolling pin.) Place them in a saucepan along with the rice. Heat over medium heat, stirring constantly, until they begin to smell toasted, 3 to 4 minutes. Add the liquid and the seasonings. Mix well. Bring to a boil, cover, reduce the heat to medium-low, and cook until all water is absorbed, 30 to 40 minutes.

Millet Loaf

SERVINGS: 4
PREPARATION TIME: 10 MINUTES
COOKING TIME: 1¼ HOURS

1¼ cups millet
4 cups tomato juice
1 medium onion,
   chopped
1 to 2 cloves garlic

½ teaspoon dried sage
½ teaspoon dried basil
½ teaspoon poultry
   seasoning

Preheat the oven to 350°F.

Place the millet in a large bowl. Place the remaining ingredients in a blender and process until smooth. Add to the millet and mix well. Pour into a shallow casserole dish. Cover and bake for 1¼ hours, or until set.

Oat-Turnip Loaf

SERVINGS: 8
PREPARATION TIME: 20 MINUTES
COOKING TIME: 1 HOUR, 25 MINUTES
RESTING TIME: 15 MINUTES

5 to 6 medium turnips
⅔ cup unsweetened
applesauce

1½ cups rolled oats
¼ cup water

Cut the turnips into large chunks. Place in a saucepan with water to cover. Cook over medium heat until tender, about 25 minutes. Drain.

Preheat the oven to 350°F.

When the turnips are cool enough to handle, peel away the tough outer skins and mash with a potato masher. Place in a bowl and add the remaining ingredients. Mix well. Press into one large (9¼ × 5¼-inch) or three small (5½ × 3½-inch) nonstick loaf pans. Bake for 1 hour, or until set. Let rest 15 minutes. Loosen the sides and invert onto a plate.

Note: This freezes well. Wrap tightly in plastic wrap. If you slice before wrapping, it will be easier to thaw and reheat in a microwave oven.

Oat-Nut Burgers

SERVINGS: 6 TO 8
PREPARATION TIME: 10 MINUTES
RESTING TIME: 20 MINUTES
COOKING TIME: 20 TO 30 MINUTES

This is a rich recipe because of the walnuts, a high-fat plant food, and the soy milk.

2 cups rolled oats
1 cup finely chopped walnuts
2 cups low-fat soy milk
1 medium onion, finely chopped

1 tablespoon soy sauce
½ teaspoon onion powder
½ teaspoon garlic powder
½ teaspoon dried sage
½ teaspoon dried thyme
¼ teaspoon dried marjoram

Mix all of the ingredients together. Let rest for 20 minutes. Form into six or eight patties. Cook on a nonstick griddle over medium heat until browned on each side, 20 to 30 minutes.

Main Dish Seitan and Tofu Dishes

Seitan

Seitan is seasoned, cooked wheat gluten. It is used as a substitute for meat. Because it is made from the protein part of the wheat, it is a high-protein food. Seitan may be purchased in most natural-food stores. It is also possible to make seitan at home. It will take a little time and work, but it is much less expensive than the commercial varieties.

You will need 8 cups of whole-wheat flour and 3 to 4 cups of water. Place the flour in a large bowl. Add the water, 1 cup at a time, until you have a kneadable dough. Turn out onto a floured board and thoroughly knead until elastic, 15 to 20 minutes. Place the dough in a bowl and cover with cold water. Let the dough rest in the water for at least 30 minutes. Then knead the dough under the water. When the water begins to turn milky from the starch, carefully pour off the water. Add new water and continue to knead. Repeat this process until the water is clear. What you are left with is raw gluten.

Let the raw gluten sit in a bowl while you prepare the seitan stock (see below). Raw gluten may be stored in the refrigerator for several days before the seasoning process.

Cut the gluten into cubes or slices. Put the gluten into the seitan stock and cook gently for 1 to 1½ hours. After cooking, the gluten is now seitan. It may be used at once or stored in the cooking liquid in the refrigerator. It will keep for about a week. To freeze the seitan, remove it from the liquid and freeze in a covered container. Freezing will not change the taste or texture of seitan. Be sure to save the seitan stock for use in soups or stews.

SEITAN STOCK

SERVINGS: MAKES 2 QUARTS
PREPARATION TIME: 10 MINUTES   COOKING TIME: 1 TO 1½ HOURS

2 quarts water
½ cup soy sauce
1 tablespoon grated fresh
ginger

1 to 2 cloves garlic, crushed
One 3- to 4-inch piece
kombu (optional; see
Note)

Combine all of the ingredients in a soup pot. Bring to a boil, cover, reduce the heat, and simmer gently. Add raw gluten to this mixture and cook gently for 1 to 1½ hours.

Note: Kombu is seaweed, usually found in natural-food stores or Asian markets.

Moroccan Seitan

SERVINGS: 6 TO 8
PREPARATION TIME: 15 MINUTES (NEED PREPARED SEITAN)
COOKING TIME: 40 MINUTES

Serve over whole grains.

3 onions, chopped
2 cloves garlic, crushed
½ cup water
One 15-ounce can whole
tomatoes, chopped, with
liquid
One 15-ounce can garbanzo
beans, rinsed and
drained
2 cups cubed seitan

2 teaspoons grated orange
zest
1 teaspoon ground
coriander
½ teaspoon ground
cinnamon
½ cup raisins
Freshly ground pepper
to taste

Place the onion, garlic, and water in a large saucepan. Sauté until the onion softens, about 10 minutes. Add the remaining ingredients, except the raisins and pepper. Cook over medium-low heat for 15 minutes. Add the raisins and continue to cook for 15 minutes longer. Season with pepper to taste.

Seitan Bourguignon

SERVINGS: 6 TO 8
PREPARATION TIME: 15 MINUTES (NEED PREPARED SEITAN)
COOKING TIME: 1 HOUR

Serve over rice, pasta, potatoes, or bread.

3 medium onions, sliced
½ pound mushrooms, sliced
½ cup water
2 cups cubed seitan
1 cup nonalcoholic red wine (see Note)
1½ cups vegetable broth (or liquid from making seitan)

⅓ cup soy sauce
¼ teaspoon dried marjoram
¼ teaspoon dried thyme
⅛ teaspoon freshly ground black pepper
2½ tablespoons cornstarch, mixed with ¼ cup water

Place the onion and mushrooms in a large pot with the water. Sauté for about 15 minutes, or until tender. Add the remaining ingredients, except the cornstarch mixture. Cover and cook over medium-low heat for about 45 minutes. Add the cornstarch mixture. Cook, stirring, until thickened.

Note: Nonalcoholic wine can be purchased at some natural-food stores and some liquor stores.

Spicy Tofu Sloppy Joes

SERVINGS: 8

PREPARATION TIME: 15 MINUTES (NOT COUNTING FREEZING
AND THAWING OF TOFU)
COOKING TIME: 20 MINUTES

*The tofu must be frozen for at least a day and then thawed before it is
used in this recipe. (See the Note below.)*

Serve this on whole-wheat buns with the garnishes of your choice.

2 cloves garlic, chopped
1 onion, chopped
1 green bell pepper,
chopped
1 pound tofu, frozen and
thawed (see Note)
½ cup soy sauce

1 tablespoon Dijon
mustard
1 tablespoon honey
2 teaspoons cider vinegar
1 to 2 teaspoons grated fresh
ginger
Dash or two cayenne

Place the garlic, onion, and green pepper in a saucepan with a
small amount of water. Cook, stirring, until the onion and green
pepper soften. Squeeze the excess water from the tofu and crumble.
Add to the saucepan, along with the remaining ingredients. Mix
well and continue to cook for 10 to 15 minutes, stirring occasionally.

Note: Tofu may be frozen in the package in which it is sold, including the liquid. Just place the unopened package in the freezer
and freeze for at least 1 day before using in this recipe. Tofu may
also be removed from the package, drained, placed in a plastic
freezer container or bag, and frozen. Freezing changes the tofu
from a soft, cheesy consistency to a chewy meatlike texture. To
thaw, remove from the freezer and let thaw at room temperature
for 6 to 8 hours. To quick-thaw, remove the tofu from the package
in which it was frozen, place in a large bowl, and cover with boiling water. This will thaw the tofu in about 1 hour. After thawing,
press out excess water.

Spicy Marinated Tofu

SERVINGS: 2 TO 4
PREPARATION TIME: 10 MINUTES, PLUS 1 HOUR MARINATING TIME
COOKING TIME: 40 MINUTES

One 14-ounce package tofu, frozen and thawed (see Note, page 269)
½ cup soy sauce
1 tablespoon honey
2 teaspoons cider vinegar
2 teaspoons dry mustard
1 to 2 teaspoons grated fresh ginger
2 teaspoons onion powder
2 cloves garlic, crushed
Dash cayenne

Cut the tofu into ¼-inch-thick strips. Combine the remaining ingredients. Lay the tofu in a medium baking dish; do not overlap the strips. Pour the marinade over the tofu. Let marinate for 1 hour.

Preheat the oven to 350°F.

Bake the tofu in the marinade for 20 minutes on the first side; turn over and bake for another 20 minutes.

Open-Face Tofu-Vegetable Patties

SERVINGS: 6
PREPARATION TIME: 30 MINUTES
COOKING TIME: 45 MINUTES

Serve on whole-wheat toast with Tangy Mushroom Sauce.

1 cup sliced mushrooms
1 bunch scallions, chopped
½ cup finely chopped cauliflower pieces
½ cup finely chopped broccoli pieces
¼ cup water
2 tablespoons soy sauce
1 pound tofu
¼ teaspoon ground turmeric
1 cup whole-wheat flour
1 teaspoon baking powder

Preheat the oven to 350°F.

Sauté the vegetables in the water and 1 tablespoon of the soy sauce until the vegetables are tender-crisp and the liquid is absorbed, about 5 minutes. Remove from the heat and set aside.

Place the tofu, remaining 1 tablespoon soy sauce, and the turmeric in a blender or food processor and carefully process until fairly smooth. Remove from the jar and place in a bowl.

Add the flour and baking powder to the tofu mixture. Then add the vegetables. Mix well and form into 6 patties, 3 inches in diameter and ½ inch thick. Place on a nonstick baking sheet.

Bake for 30 minutes; turn over and bake for 15 minutes longer.

Tofu Stir-"Fry"

SERVINGS: 4 TO 6
PREPARATION TIME: 15 MINUTES
COOKING TIME: 7 TO 10 MINUTES

Serve over brown rice.

⅓ cup water
3 tablespoons soy sauce
2 cloves garlic, minced
1½ teaspoons grated fresh ginger
½ pound firm tofu, cut into strips
2 small zucchini, sliced
3 small yellow squash, sliced

½ pound snow peas, trimmed
1 small baby bok choy, sliced
1 bunch scallions, sliced into 1-inch pieces
¼ pound oyster mushrooms, sliced
½ cup bean sprouts

Combine the water, soy sauce, garlic, and ginger in a wok or large pan and bring to a boil.

Add the tofu, zucchini, squash, snow peas, and bok choy to the pan. Sauté for 4 to 5 minutes. Add the scallions, mushrooms, and bean sprouts. Sauté for another 3 to 5 minutes.

Spicy Tofu Burgers

SERVINGS: 8
PREPARATION TIME: 15 MINUTES
COOKING TIME: 30 MINUTES

Serve on whole-wheat buns with your favorite garnishes.

1 pound firm tofu, drained
1½ cup rolled oats
2 tablespoons soy sauce
1 tablespoon Worcestershire
  sauce
1 tablespoon Dijon mustard
¼ teaspoon freshly ground
  black pepper

¼ teaspoon garlic powder
¼ teaspoon onion powder
1 teaspoon grated fresh
  ginger (optional)
2 tablespoons minced fresh
  parsley (optional)

Preheat the oven to 350°F.

Place the tofu in a large bowl and mash with a potato masher. Add the remaining ingredients and stir until well combined. Moisten your hands. Shape into eight patties and place on a nonstick baking sheet. Bake for 20 minutes on the first side; turn over and bake an additional 10 minutes. Remove from the oven and cool on a rack.

Reheat by placing under the broiler or in the microwave for a few minutes.

Calzones

SERVINGS: 6

PREPARATION TIME: 1½ HOURS   COOKING TIME: 30 MINUTES

Leftover stews, bean dishes, and Mexican foods would also make excellent calzone fillings.

> 1 recipe Pizza Crust
> (page 228)

FILLING

> 1 pound spinach, washed   1 tablespoon chopped
>   and trimmed   fresh basil
> ½ cup chopped onion   ¼ cup grated soy
> 2 cloves garlic, crushed   Parmesan cheese
> 1 to 2 zucchini, chopped   (optional)
> 1 pound tofu, mashed   Freshly ground pepper
> 1 tablespoon soy sauce   to taste

Prepare the crust as directed, through the rising. While the dough is rising, prepare the filling.

Place the washed spinach in a large pan, using only the water clinging to the leaves for moisture. Cook, stirring, over low heat until wilted, about 1 minute. Remove the spinach from the pan and drain well. Add the onion, garlic, and zucchini to the pan with a small amount of water. Cook for 5 minutes. Remove from the pan and drain.

Combine all of the filling ingredients in a bowl and set aside. Preheat the oven to 375°F.

Remove the dough from the bowl and knead for a couple of minutes. Divide it into six equal pieces. Roll each piece into a circle about 7 to 8 inches in diameter and between ⅛ and ¼ inch thick. Place about ½ to ¾ cup of the filling on one half of each circle, leaving a small edge for sealing. Brush the edges with water and fold the circle over, making a half-circle. Press the edges together firmly with a fork to seal.

Place the calzones on a nonstick baking tray. Prick the top of each calzone several times with a fork to let steam escape. Bake for 30 minutes, or until golden brown.

Main Dish Legumes

Spicy Rice and Beans

SERVINGS: 4 TO 6
PREPARATION TIME: 10 MINUTES
COOKING TIME: 1 HOUR

3 cups water
1½ cups long-grain brown
  rice
One 19-ounce can kidney
  beans, rinsed and
  drained

2 cups chopped onion
1 cup mild salsa
1 teaspoon ground cumin
One 16-ounce can whole
  tomatoes, chopped

Bring the water to a boil. Stir in the rice. When the liquid boils again, stir in the kidney beans, onion, salsa, and cumin; return to a boil. Reduce the heat to low. Cover and simmer for 45 minutes. Remove from the heat and stir in the tomatoes. Let stand, covered, for 5 minutes.

Three-Bean Pilaf

SERVINGS: 6 TO 8
PREPARATION TIME: 15 MINUTES
COOKING TIME: 50 MINUTES
RESTING TIME: 15 MINUTES

2 tablespoons water
1 medium onion, chopped
2 cups long-grain brown rice
4 cups vegetable broth or water
One 15-ounce can kidney beans, drained and rinsed
One 15-ounce can garbanzo beans, drained and rinsed
One 15-ounce can black beans, drained and rinsed
One 15-ounce can stewed tomatoes
One 4-ounce can chopped green chilies
2 cups frozen corn kernels

Heat the water in a large heavy saucepan. Add the onion and cook for 2 to 3 minutes, until the onion softens. Add the rice, vegetable broth, canned beans, and the tomatoes. Stir and bring the mixture to a boil. Reduce the heat until the mixture boils gently. Cover and simmer for 30 minutes.

Stir in the chilies and corn. Cover and cook for 15 minutes longer. Let rest for 15 minutes before serving.

DHB's Pasta Fazoola

DHB are the initials of the woman who sent us this recipe. This is one of her family's favorites.

SERVINGS: 6
PREPARATION TIME: 20 MINUTES
COOKING TIME: 45 MINUTES

Serve with hot-pepper flakes or hot sauce to taste.

One 16-ounce can kidney
    beans, drained and
    rinsed
One 32-ounce can whole
    tomatoes, chopped
1 clove garlic, minced
1 onion, chopped
½ cup chopped celery
    Freshly ground pepper
    to taste

½ pound elbow macaroni
3 medium tomatoes,
    chopped
1 jalapeño pepper,
    chopped
2 leaves Swiss chard
    (stalks removed), sliced
    into ¼-inch pieces

Place the kidney beans, canned tomatoes, garlic, onion, celery, and pepper in a large saucepan. Cook over low heat for 30 minutes.

Cook elbow macaroni in boiling water until just tender, 8 to 10 minutes. Add to the bean and tomato mixture. Add the fresh tomatoes, Swiss chard, and jalapeño pepper. Heat through thoroughly.

Note: The bean-tomato mixture may be cooked ahead and refrigerated. After cooking the pasta, reheat the bean-tomato mixture and proceed as directed.

Indian Garbanzo and Tomato Stew

SERVINGS: 4 TO 6
PREPARATION TIME: 30 MINUTES (NEED COOKED BEANS)
COOKING TIME: 50 MINUTES

This is excellent served over brown basmati rice.

⅓ cup water
1 large onion, quartered and thinly sliced
One 1-inch piece fresh ginger, peeled and minced
2 cloves garlic, peeled and minced
1 teaspoon *each* coriander seeds, cumin seeds, and black mustard seeds

1 teaspoon curry powder
1½ pounds tomatoes, seeded and pureed
1 green bell pepper, cut into ½-inch dice
1 red bell pepper, cut into ½-inch dice
3 cups cooked garbanzo beans
1 tablespoon Garam Masala (recipe follows)

Place the water in a medium saucepan. Sauté the onion, ginger, garlic, seeds, and curry powder, over medium-low heat, stirring frequently, until the onion is tender, about 10 minutes. Add the tomatoes and simmer, uncovered, for 10 minutes. Add the peppers and garbanzos. Reduce the heat, cover, and simmer for 30 minutes, stirring occasionally. If too thin, cook uncovered to a thick stew consistency. Stir in the garam masala and serve.

GARAM MASALA

SERVINGS: MAKES 3 TABLESPOONS

4 teaspoons ground coriander
2 teaspoons ground cumin
1 teaspoon freshly ground black pepper

1 teaspoon ground cloves
1 teaspoon ground cinnamon

Mix all of the ingredients together and store in a tightly covered jar.

Moroccan Chick-Peas

SERVINGS: 6

PREPARATION TIME: 10 MINUTES, PLUS 1 HOUR STANDING TIME

COOKING TIME: 2½ TO 3 HOURS

The woman who sent me this recipe adapted it from a Moroccan chicken recipe. She claims it looks better now because the chicken fat–turmeric combination made green grease.

Serve alone or over rice or other whole grains.

2 cups dried chick-peas (garbanzo beans)	1 cinnamon stick
2 quarts cold water	1 teaspoon ground ginger
1 bay leaf	1 teaspoon ground turmeric
2 cloves garlic, crushed	¼ teaspoon freshly ground black pepper
1 cup chopped onion	½ to ¾ cup raisins (to taste)
2 tablespoons chopped fresh parsley	

Pick over the chick-peas. Rinse. Place them in a large soup pot and add water to cover. Bring to a boil. Boil for 2 minutes, remove from the heat, cover, and let stand for 1 hour. Pour off the water.

Add the 2 quarts of cold water and the bay leaf. Bring to a boil, reduce the heat, cover, and cook over medium heat for 1½ hours.

Add the remaining ingredients, except the raisins. Continue to cook until the chick-peas are tender, at least 1 hour longer. Add the raisins and cook for 15 minutes more. Remove the bay leaf and cinnamon stick.

Yaknit El Batingann
(Eggplant and Garbanzo Stew)

SERVINGS: 6

PREPARATION TIME: 25 MINUTES, PLUS OVERNIGHT SOAKING

COOKING TIME: 3½ TO 4 HOURS FOR GARBANZOS, 30 MINUTES FOR STEW

This is a typical Middle Eastern vegetable dish. Serve with Rice and Noodle Pilaf and Adas Bi Sabaanikh.

2 cups dried garbanzo beans

10 cups water

1 large eggplant, cut into 1-inch cubes

2 potatoes, peeled and cut into 1-inch cubes

1 large onion, chopped

2 leeks, washed and chopped

2 to 3 cloves garlic, crushed

2 cups reserved garbanzo stock

One 15-ounce can stewed tomatoes

¼ cup chopped fresh parsley

¼ teaspoon black pepper

¼ cup tomato paste

¼ cup fresh lemon juice

Place the garbanzo beans and water in a large pot. Bring to a boil, cover, and cook over medium heat until the beans are tender, about 4 hours. Beans may also be soaked overnight then cooked according to the same directions, although cooking time should be reduced by ½ hour. Remove from the heat and drain, reserving the stock for later use. Set aside.

Preheat the broiler.

Place the eggplant on a nonstick baking tray. Place under the broiler about 8 inches from the heat and broil for about 5 minutes. Watch carefully to make sure the eggplant doesn't burn. Set aside.

Place the potatoes, onion, leeks, and garlic in a pot with the 2 cups of garbanzo stock. Bring to a boil, cover, and cook over medium-low heat for about 15 minutes. Add the reserved eggplant and continue to cook for another 5 to 10 minutes. Add the cooked garbanzos, the tomatoes, parsley, pepper, and tomato paste. Mix well. Cook for an additional 5 minutes. Add the lemon juice. Mix in well and serve at once.

Variations: This recipe can easily be varied to suit your own tastes. Some suggestions: Substitute 2 cups of any other dried bean for the garbanzo beans. Substitute broccoli for eggplant. Do not broil the broccoli; just add it to the stew in place of the eggplant.

Garbanzo-Broccoli Stew

SERVINGS: 4 TO 6
PREPARATION TIME: 30 MINUTES, PLUS OVERNIGHT SOAKING
COOKING TIME: 3 HOURS

1 cup dried garbanzo beans
7 cups vegetable broth (page 132)
1 medium onion, coarsely chopped
2 medium sweet potatoes, chunked
1 large carrot, scrubbed and sliced
1 stalk celery, sliced
1 leek, washed, halved lengthwise, and cut into 1½-inch slices

1 jalapeño pepper, scored and left whole (optional)
2 cups broccoli pieces (florets and stalk)
1 tablespoon fresh lemon juice
1 teaspoon ground coriander
1½ teaspoons ground cumin

Soak the beans overnight in water to cover. Drain and rinse. Put the beans in a large pot with the vegetable broth. Bring to a boil. Reduce the heat and simmer, covered for 2½ hours.

Add the onion, sweet potato, carrot, celery, leek, and hot pepper. Continue simmering for 15 minutes. Add the remaining ingredients. Simmer for 15 minutes longer. Discard the pepper and serve.

Falafel

SERVINGS: 8
PREPARATION TIME: 35 MINUTES
COOKING TIME: 15 MINUTES

These can be messy to eat, but they are a delicious, easy meal.

1 package falafel mix
(Fantastic Foods or
Casbah)
1¼ cups water
8 whole-wheat pita breads
1 tomato, sliced
1 small cucumber, sliced

1 bunch scallions, chopped
1½ cups torn lettuce leaves
1 cup mung bean sprouts
(optional)
1 recipe Tahini Sauce (see
page 341)

Pour the falafel mix into a bowl. Mix with the water and let rest for
15 minutes.

Cut the pita breads through the centers to form two "pockets."
Set aside. Assemble all of the remaining ingredients and place in
separate bowls. Set aside.

Heat a nonstick griddle over medium heat. Form the falafel
mixture into patties about the size of the pita "pockets." Place the
patties on the griddle and cook for 5 to 7½ minutes on each side,
until slightly brown. Remove from the griddle and place on a serving platter.

To assemble: Place one falafel patty into a pita "pocket." Stuff
with tomato, cucumber, scallions, lettuce, and sprouts. Spoon some
Tahini Sauce over the filling and eat, using your fingers. Be prepared for drips.

Note: For a lower-fat version, omit the Tahini Sauce and use some
nonfat salad dressing instead.

Garbanzo Shepherd's Pie

SERVINGS: 6 TO 8

PREPARATION TIME: 35 MINUTES (NEED COOKED BEANS)

COOKING TIME: 50 MINUTES

1 large onion, chopped
½ pound mushrooms, chopped
½ cup water
1½ cups diced carrot
¾ cup diced celery
½ bunch spinach, washed and trimmed (about 2 cups)
2 cups low-fat soy milk
1 tablespoon soy sauce
½ tablespoon Parsley Patch seasoning, general blend
¼ teaspoon garlic powder
2 tablespoons cornstarch, mixed with ¼ cup cold water
2 cups cooked garbanzo beans
1½ cups frozen green peas, thawed
Mashed potatoes (recipe follows)
Paprika

Preheat the oven to 325°F.

Place the onion and mushrooms in a large pot with the water. Cook, stirring, for 5 minutes. Add the carrot and celery, and continue to cook, stirring frequently, until the carrot and celery are tender, about 10 minutes. Add the spinach, cover, and steam until wilted, about 1 minute. Remove from the heat.

In a separate saucepan, mix the soy milk with the soy sauce, Parsley Patch, and garlic powder. Add the cornstarch mixture and cook, stirring, until the mixture boils and thickens. Add to the vegetable mixture, then stir in the garbanzos and peas.

Spoon into six to eight individual casserole dishes. Top with mashed potatoes and sprinkle with paprika. Bake for 30 minutes, or until golden.

MASHED POTATOES

4 large potatoes, peeled and diced
1 cup low-fat soy milk
¼ teaspoon onion powder

Steam the potatoes over boiling water for 15 minutes. Place in a bowl; add the soy milk and onion powder. Mash with a potato masher until smooth.

Easy Baked Beans

SERVINGS: 8
PREPARATION TIME: 15 MINUTES
COOKING TIME: 2½ TO 3 HOURS

1½ cups navy beans
8 cups water
1 bay leaf
½ cup finely chopped onion
½ cup finely chopped green
  bell pepper

1 teaspoon minced garlic
½ cup tomato puree
3 tablespoons molasses
1 tablespoon fresh lemon
  juice

Place the beans and water in a large pot, along with the bay leaf, onion, green pepper, and garlic. Cover and cook until the beans are tender, 1½ to 2 hours. Remove from the heat and drain, reserving the cooking liquid. Remove the bay leaf.

Preheat the oven to 300°F.

Transfer the cooked beans and vegetables to a casserole dish with a cover. Add the remaining ingredients and 1 cup of the reserved cooking liquid. Mix well. Bake, covered, for 1 hour. Stir occasionally during baking and add a little more cooking liquid if needed to keep the beans moist.

Smashed Beans

SERVINGS: MAKES ABOUT 6 CUPS
PREPARATION TIME: 10 MINUTES, PLUS OVERNIGHT SOAKING
COOKING TIME: 3 TO 4 HOURS (OR ALL DAY IN A SLOW COOKER)

Use for bean nachos, tacos, burritos, casseroles, or dips.

2 cups pinto beans
8 cups water
½ teaspoon onion
powder

½ teaspoon garlic powder
½ to 1 cup mild or spicy salsa

Place the beans in a large pot with the water. Bring to a boil, cover, reduce the heat, and cook until tender, 3 to 4 hours. (To reduce the cooking time, soak the beans overnight in the water. Then proceed as directed, reducing cooking time by ½ hour.) Drain, reserving the cooking liquid.

Mash the beans, using a hand masher, electric beater, or food processor. Return to the pan. Add the spices, a little of the reserved cooking liquid, and the salsa, stirring until the beans have a softened, smashed consistency. Heat through to blend the flavors.

Cuban Black Beans

SERVINGS: 8

PREPARATION TIME: 20 MINUTES, PLUS OVERNIGHT SOAKING

COOKING TIME: 2 HOURS, 45 MINUTES

Serve over rice or other whole grains or in a bowl by itself.

1 pound black beans
10½ cups water
1 green bell pepper, cut in half
1 onion, finely chopped
1 green bell pepper, finely chopped
4 cloves garlic, pressed
1 tablespoon Mrs. Dash seasoning
1 tablespoon honey
1 bay leaf
¼ teaspoon dried oregano
2 tablespoons cider vinegar

Soak the beans overnight in water to cover. Drain. Place the beans, 10 cups water, and green-pepper halves in a large pot. Cook over medium heat until the green pepper is soft, about 45 minutes. Remove the green pepper and discard.

Meanwhile, sauté the onion, chopped green pepper, and garlic in the remaining ½ cup water until soft, 15 to 20 minutes. Add 1 cup of the cooked beans; mash the beans and vegetables with a potato masher. Add to the large pot of beans, along with the Mrs. Dash, honey, bay leaf, and oregano. Cover and cook over low heat for 1 hour. Add the vinegar and continue to cook for another hour. If the mixture seems too thin, remove the cover during the last hour of cooking.

Confetti Beans

SERVINGS: 6
PREPARATION TIME: 15 MINUTES (NEED COOKED BEANS)
COOKING TIME: 10 MINUTES

These beans can be served any number of ways. Try them rolled up in burrito shells, on burger buns, or over grains, pasta, or baked potatoes.

1 onion, chopped
2 red or green bell
  peppers, chopped
1 to 2 cloves garlic, pressed
¼ cup water
3 cups cooked beans
  (pinto, black, garbanzo,
  etc.)
2 cups frozen corn
  kernels

One 15-ounce can stewed
  tomatoes (try Cajun,
  Mexican, or Italian)
1 tablespoon chili
  powder
Freshly ground black
  pepper to taste

Sauté the onion, bell pepper, and garlic in the water until softened, 4 to 5 minutes. Add the remaining ingredients, cover, and cook over low heat for another 5 minutes.

Ranch-Style Beans

SERVINGS: 6 TO 8
PREPARATION TIME: 10 MINUTES   COOKING TIME: 20 MINUTES

½ cup chopped onion
½ cup chopped green bell
  pepper
½ cup water
Two 16-ounce cans vegetarian
  oil-free baked beans
One 15-ounce can kidney
  beans, drained and rinsed

One 8-ounce can tomato
  sauce
¼ cup molasses
2 tablespoons prepared
  mustard

Place the onion and green pepper in a medium saucepan with the water. Cook, stirring, for 5 minutes. Add the remaining ingredients and simmer over low heat, uncovered, for 15 minutes, stirring occasionally.

Spicy Red Beans

SERVINGS: 8 TO 10
PREPARATION TIME: 15 MINUTES
COOKING TIME: 3 HOURS (8 TO 10 HOURS IN A SLOW COOKER)

Serve over brown rice.

2 cups red beans
3 onions, chopped
8 cloves garlic, crushed
One 4-ounce can chopped green chilies
1 jalapeño pepper, seeded and chopped (optional)
One 16-ounce can whole tomatoes, chopped with liquid
One 15-ounce can tomato sauce
2 stalks celery, chopped
6 cups water
2 tablespoons chopped fresh parsley

2 tablespoons paprika
2 teaspoons white pepper
6 bay leaves
1 teaspoon dried oregano
1 teaspoon dried rosemary
1 teaspoon dried thyme
1 teaspoon dried marjoram
1 teaspoon dried savory
1 teaspoon dried tarragon
1 teaspoon dried basil
1 teaspoon Tabasco (or more to taste)

Combine all of the ingredients in a large pot or slow cooker. Simmer over medium-low heat until the beans are tender. This will take about 3 hours on top of the stove and 8 to 10 hours on the high setting of a slow cooker.

Note: This recipe freezes well in a tightly covered container. Thaw overnight in the refrigerator and reheat on top of the stove or in the microwave.

McDougall's Favorite Bean Burritos

SERVINGS: 10 TO 12
PREPARATION TIME: 20 MINUTES
COOKING TIME: 3 TO 4 HOURS

2 cups pinto beans	1 to 2 cups cooked brown
8 cups water	rice (optional)
½ to 1 cup mild salsa	Additional salsa
2 tomatoes, chopped	(spicy or mild,
1 bunch scallions,	depending on your
chopped	taste)
1 cup alfalfa sprouts	10 to 12 whole-wheat tortillas
2 cups shredded lettuce	

Place the beans in a large pot with the water. Bring to a boil, cover, reduce the heat slightly to avoid a boilover, and cook until tender, 3 to 4 hours (depending on the age of the beans and how tender you like them). Drain, reserving the cooking liquid.

Mash the beans with a hand masher or portable electric beater. (This can also be done in your food processor.) Add a little of the bean cooking liquid and the mild salsa, until the beans achieve a soft, moist consistency.

To serve, place all of the ingredients in separate bowls, except the tortillas. Let each person make his or her own tortilla by layering on the ingredients of choice. For instance: Spread a line of beans down the center of a tortilla, spread some rice over the beans, if desired, then add some tomato, scallions, sprouts, and lettuce. Spoon a little of your favorite salsa over all of this, roll up the tortilla, and either place on a plate and eat it using a fork or pick it up and eat it using your fingers.

Spicy Mung Bean Roll-Ups

SERVINGS: 12
PREPARATION TIME: 5 MINUTES
COOKING TIME: 1 HOUR

This also makes a delicious sandwich spread.

2 cups skinned mung beans
(see Note)
4½ cups water
1 tablespoon soy sauce
1 tablespoon curry powder

¼ teaspoon Thai chili
powder (optional; see
Note)
12 whole-wheat tortillas

Pick over the beans and discard any stones. Place the beans and water in a medium pot. Bring to a boil, reduce the heat to low, cover, and cook for 30 minutes. Add the seasonings and continue to cook for another 30 minutes, or until the mixture has thickened.

To serve, place the tortillas next to the bean mixture. Let each diner make his or her own roll-up by placing a line of the beans down the center of the tortilla, then rolling it up and eating with the fingers.

Note: Skinned mung beans and Thai chili powder can be found in many Oriental markets.

Variation: Serve garnishes to add to the filling before rolling up and eating. Some examples: chopped scallion, chopped fresh parsley or cilantro, bean sprouts, alfalfa sprouts.

Bean-Corn Enchiladas

SERVINGS: 8

PREPARATION TIME: 30 MINUTES (NEED COOKED BEANS)

COOKING TIME: 30 MINUTES

½ cup chopped green bell pepper
½ cup chopped scallion
⅓ cup water
2 cups cooked pinto beans
1 cup frozen corn kernels
3 teaspoons diced green chilies (canned)

2 teaspoons minced garlic
2 teaspoons ground cumin
16 corn tortillas
1 recipe Enchilada Sauce (page 336)
Several sprigs fresh cilantro

Sauté the green pepper and scallion in the water until softened, about 5 minutes.

Mix the beans, corn, chilies, garlic, and cumin in a bowl. Add the sautéed vegetables. Mix well.

Preheat the oven to 375°F.

Steam the tortillas for 1 minute or wrap them in a cloth and heat in the microwave on high for 1 minute. Dip the tortillas in heated Enchilada Sauce, being careful not to soak them. Spoon about ¼ cup of the bean mixture on each, and roll up.

Place on a nonstick 13 × 9-inch baking dish, seam side down. Bake for 15 to 20 minutes, or until bubbly. Remove from the oven and cover with the remaining sauce. Garnish with cilantro. Serve at once.

Black Bean Burritos

SERVINGS: 6 TO 8

PREPARATION TIME: 10 MINUTES (NEED COOKED BEANS)

COOKING TIME: 10 MINUTES

2 cups cooked black beans
¼ cup chopped onion
¼ cup fresh salsa

1 tomato, chopped
3 scallions, chopped
8 whole-wheat tortillas

Place the beans, onion, and ¼ cup of salsa in a saucepan and heat through.

Place a line of bean mixture down the center of a tortilla. Add tomato and scallions and roll up.

Variation: Add 2 cups cooked brown rice and an extra ½ cup of salsa to the saucepan with the beans and heat through. Serve as above.

Four-Bean Enchiladas

SERVINGS: 8

PREPARATION TIME: 20 MINUTES (NEED PREPARED ENCHILADA SAUCE)

COOKING TIME: 30 MINUTES

One 15-ounce can kidney beans, rinsed and drained

One 15-ounce can garbanzo beans, rinsed and drained

One 15-ounce can pinto beans, rinsed and drained

One 15-ounce can black beans, rinsed and drained

1½ cups salsa

16 fresh soft corn tortillas

2½ cups Enchilada Sauce (page 336)

½ cup chopped scallion

Preheat the oven to 350°F.

Combine the beans and the salsa in a medium bowl.

Spread about ⅓ cup of the bean mixture down the center of a tortilla. Roll up and place, seam-side down, in an oblong nonstick baking dish that has ½ cup of the Enchilada Sauce spread over the bottom. Repeat until all of the tortillas are filled. Pour the rest of the sauce over the tortillas and sprinkle with the scallion.

Cover with parchment paper, then cover with foil, wrapping the edges tightly. Bake for 30 minutes.

Bean Tacos

SERVINGS: 8

PREPARATION TIME: 20 MINUTES (NEED PREPARED BEANS)

COOKING TIME: 5 TO 7 MINUTES

8 soft corn tortillas	1 to 2 tomatoes, chopped
1 recipe for prepared beans (see Lentil Enchiladas, below; Black Bean Burritos, page 290; or Smashed Beans, page 284)	1 bunch scallions, chopped
	2 cups shredded iceberg lettuce
	Salsa

Preheat the oven to 450°F.

To make taco shells, invert a jelly-roll pan in the center of a cookie sheet. Fold each tortilla over the edge of the pan in a taco shape. Bake for 5 to 7 minutes, or until crisp. (If you do not have a jelly-roll pan, use anything you can think of to hold the tortillas in a taco shape while they are baking.

Heat the beans thoroughly over low heat. To assemble, put some beans in the bottom of the taco shell, then layer on the remaining ingredients. Repeat until all of the ingredients are used up.

Lentil Enchiladas

SERVINGS: 8 TO 12

PREPARATION TIME: 10 MINUTES   COOKING TIME: 45 MINUTES

1 cup lentils	Chopped tomato for garnish (optional)
3 cups water	
1 small onion, chopped	Chopped scallion for garnish (optional)
1 clove garlic, crushed	
¼ cup salsa	Green Enchilada Sauce (page 338)
8 to 12 soft corn tortillas	

Place the lentils, water, onion, and garlic in a saucepan. Bring to a boil, reduce the heat, and cook until the lentils are mushy, about 45 minutes. Drain off any excess water. Add the salsa and mix in well.

Place a line of the lentils down the center of each tortilla. Add garnishes if desired and roll up. Cover with Green Enchilada Sauce. Serve hot.

Baked Lentil Burritos with Green Enchilada Sauce

SERVINGS: 6 TO 10
PREPARATION TIME: 15 MINUTES (NEED COOKED LENTILS AND SAUCE)
COOKING TIME: 45 MINUTES

3 cups Green Enchilada
  Sauce (page 338)
10 flour tortillas

3 cups lentil mix (from
  Lentil Enchiladas,
  opposite page)

Preheat the oven to 350°F.

Place 1 cup of the sauce in the bottom of a nonstick oblong 11¾ × 7½-inch casserole.

Place a line of the lentil mixture down the center of each tortilla. Roll them up and place them, seam-sides down, in the casserole dish.

Pour the remaining 2 cups of sauce over the burritos. Cover and bake for 45 minutes.

Tortilla Casserole

SERVINGS: 4
PREPARATION TIME: 10 MINUTES (NEED COOKED BEANS AND CHIPS)
COOKING TIME: 45 MINUTES

1 7-ounce package oil-free
tortilla chips (or make
your own; see page 126)
4 cups Smashed Beans (page
284)

2 cups salsa
½ cup grated soy cheddar
cheese

Preheat the oven to 350°F.

Line the bottom of an oblong 11 × 9-inch casserole dish with the tortilla chips. Spread the beans over the chips, then the salsa. Sprinkle with the cheese.

Bake, covered, for 45 minutes, or until the cheese is melted and bubbly.

Lentil Chili and Cornbread Casserole

SERVINGS: 8
PREPARATION TIME: 40 MINUTES
COOKING TIME: 1½ HOURS

CHILI

2 onions, chopped
3 tablespoons minced
garlic
¾ cup water
¼ cup chili powder
1 tablespoon ground
cumin
2 teaspoons paprika
1 teaspoon dried thyme
½ teaspoon dried oregano

2 bay leaves
5 cups vegetable broth
(page 132) or water
2 cups lentils
One 15- to 16-ounce can
whole tomatoes,
chopped
2 medium green bell
peppers, chopped
2 stalks celery, chopped

CORNBREAD CRUST

1½ cups cornmeal	2 teaspoons Ener-G Egg
½ cup whole-wheat	Replacer, beaten until
flour	frothy with ¼ cup water
3 teaspoons baking	1 tablespoon honey
powder	1¼ cups warm water

Cook the onion and garlic in the water in a large pot until the onion is soft, 5 to 7 minutes. Add all of the seasonings and cook, stirring, for 2 to 3 minutes. Add the vegetable stock or water and bring to a boil. Add the lentils, cover partially, reduce the heat, and simmer for 40 minutes, stirring occasionally. Add the tomatoes, green pepper, and celery. Simmer, uncovered, for 20 minutes. Spoon into eight single-serving casserole dishes, or spoon into an 11 × 9-inch casserole dish. Discard the bay leaves. Set aside.

Preheat the oven to 375°F.

Combine the cornmeal, flour, and baking powder. In a separate bowl, combine the Egg Replacer mixture, honey, and water; add to the dry ingredients, stirring until just combined.

Spoon approximately 3 tablespoons of crust mixture on top of the lentils in each small casserole or spread over the top in the large casserole. Bake single-serving casseroles for 20 minutes, the large single casserole for 30 minutes, until heated through.

Light Lentil Loaf

SERVINGS: 6 TO 8
PREPARATION TIME: 20 MINUTES (NEED COOKED RICE AND LENTILS)
COOKING TIME: 1 HOUR, 10 MINUTES

2½ cups finely chopped onion
2 cups grated carrot
5 cloves garlic, diced
¼ cup vegetable broth (page 132) or water
2 cups cooked short-grain brown rice
2 cups cooked lentils, mashed

2 cups rolled oats
2 tablespoons dark miso (traditional or red)
1 tablespoon soy sauce
2 tablespoons hot vegetable broth (page 132) or water
½ cup finely chopped fresh parsley
1 tablespoon dried sage
1 teaspoon celery seed

Preheat the oven to 350°F.

Sauté the onion, carrot, and garlic in the ¼ cup stock or water for 10 minutes. Mix with the rice, lentils, and oats. Mix the miso and soy sauce with the 2 tablespoons hot stock or water to dissolve. Add to the mixture. Add the parsley, sage, and celery seed. Mix until all of the ingredients are combined. Pack into a nonstick loaf pan and bake for 1 hour, or until firm.

Slide thin, sharp knife between the loaf and the pan. Place a serving plate on top and turn over (quickly), letting the loaf drop out onto the plate. Serve with the sauce of your choice.

Note: This may also be made into burgers. Just form into six to eight patties and bake on a nonstick baking sheet for 20 minutes on each side.

Savory Lentils

SERVINGS: 6 TO 8
PREPARATION TIME: 25 MINUTES
COOKING TIME: 2 HOURS

Excellent over mashed potatoes or whole-wheat toast.

One 12-ounce package
lentils
4 cups water
1 clove garlic, minced
1 onion, chopped
3 to 4 scallions, chopped
1 to 2 stalks celery, chopped

¼ cup soy sauce
⅓ cup balsamic vinegar
One 6-ounce can tomato
paste
1 teaspoon Dijon mustard
Freshly ground black
pepper to taste

Place the lentils in a large pot and cover with the water. Bring to a boil, cover, reduce the heat, and simmer for 1 hour.

Sauté the garlic, onion, scallions, and celery in ⅓ cup water until soft. Add to the cooked lentils, along with the soy sauce, vinegar, tomato paste, and mustard. Add freshly ground black pepper to taste. Continue to simmer for 1 hour more, covered for a souplike consistency, uncovered for a gravylike consistency.

Slow-Cooked Black Beans and Prunes

SERVINGS: 6 TO 8
PREPARATION TIME: 15 MINUTES, PLUS OVERNIGHT SOAKING
COOKING TIME: 10 TO 12 HOURS OR 6 TO 8 HOURS IN A SLOW COOKER

Serve over brown rice or another whole grain.

2½ cups black beans
6 cups water
2 onions, chopped
3 tablespoons soy sauce
1½ cups pitted prunes
One 28-ounce can whole
tomatoes, diced or sliced

2 cloves garlic, pressed
2 tablespoons honey
1 tablespoon chili powder
1 teaspoon dry mustard
3 tablespoons catsup

Soak the beans overnight in the water. Place all of the ingredients in a slow cooker. Cook on low for 10 to 12 hours or on high for 6 to 8 hours.

Note: This freezes well in a tightly covered container. Thaw overnight in the refrigerator and reheat on top of the stove or in the microwave.

Slow-Cooked Baby Lima Beans

SERVINGS: 6 TO 8
PREPARATION TIME: 10 MINUTES, PLUS OVERNIGHT SOAKING
COOKING TIME: 8 TO 10 HOURS IN A SLOW COOKER

Serve over whole grains or potatoes, or in a bowl by itself.

2 pounds baby lima beans
One 2-pound can stewed tomatoes
One 1-pound can tomato sauce
2 large onions, coarsely chopped

Freshly ground black pepper to taste
4 tablespoons brown sugar
2 or 3 large bay leaves

Cover the beans with water and soak overnight. Place all of the ingredients in a slow cooker and cook all day on low heat. If a thicker stew is desired, remove the lid of the slow cooker for the last hour or so and stir occasionally, or thicken with a small amount of cornstarch mixed in cold water.

Beanburgers

SERVINGS: 4
PREPARATION TIME: 15 MINUTES
COOKING TIME: 10 MINUTES

One 15-ounce can kidney
  beans, rinsed and
  drained
1 small onion, chopped
One 8-ounce can tomato
  sauce
  Whole-wheat bread
  crumbs (optional)

¼ teaspoon dried basil
¼ teaspoon dried
  marjoram
¼ teaspoon dried thyme
⅛ teaspoon black pepper
½ teaspoon garlic powder

Preheat the broiler.

Mash the beans. Mix in the onion and one-quarter to one-half of the tomato sauce, until the mixture has the consistency of a hamburger. (Whole-grain bread crumbs may be added to achieve the desired consistency.) Add the seasonings. Shape into four patties.

Place under the broiler and cook until lightly browned, about 5 minutes on each side. Near the end of broiling, spread the leftover tomato sauce over the patties. These may also be fried in a nonstick frying pan over medium heat for about 5 minutes on each side.

Lentil Patties

SERVINGS: 4
PREPARATION TIME: 20 MINUTES (NEED COOKED LENTILS AND POTATOES)
COOKING TIME: 40 MINUTES

Serve on whole-wheat burger buns with your favorite garnishes.

¼ cup minced onion
1 clove garlic, minced
2 tablespoons water
1 cup cooked lentils
1 cup chopped boiled
potatoes
2 tablespoons minced fresh
parsley

1 teaspoon minced fresh
basil
1 teaspoon paprika
1 teaspoon onion powder
1 teaspoon dried dill
Dash cayenne

Preheat the oven to 350°F.

Sauté the onion and garlic in the water for about 3 minutes, or until soft. Combine the lentils and potatoes in a large bowl and mash together well. Add all of the other ingredients to the lentil-potato mixture and stir until well mixed.

Form into four patties and place on a nonstick baking sheet. Bake for 20 minutes; turn over and bake for an additional 20 minutes.

Holiday Recipes

Holiday Vegebird with Dressing and Gravy

SERVINGS: 12

PREPARATION TIME: 2 HOURS (NEED COOKED RICE)

COOKING TIME: 45 MINUTES FOR RICE; 45 MINUTES FOR VEGEBIRD;

1 HOUR FOR DRESSING

The person who sent this recipe wrote, "This recipe is time consuming, but well worth it to have a meatless holiday meal. I make the dressing one day and the vegebird the next, and bake it the next day. It turns out fine and smells like Thanksgiving. The leftovers freeze well, except for the gravy."

Start cooking the rice for the vegebird before beginning the dressing.

DRESSING

7 cups whole-grain bread, in pieces

2 cups hot water

¾ cup water

½ cup diced onion

1¼ cups diced celery

¾ cup water

1 teaspoon Ener-G Egg Replacer, beaten until frothy with 2 tablespoons water

½ teaspoon dried thyme

2 teaspoons dried sage

2 teaspoons Special Seasoning (page 304)

VEGEBIRD

4 cups cooked brown rice

1½ cups finely chopped onion

3 cups ground pecans (1 pound = 3½ cups ground)

2 teaspoons garlic powder

2 teaspoons onion powder

2 teaspoons Special Seasoning (page 304)

GRAVY

¼ cup whole-wheat flour	1 teaspoon garlic powder
4 cups warm water	⅛ teaspoon freshly ground
2 tablespoons raw cashew	black pepper
pieces, rinsed	1½ teaspoons poultry
1 tablespoon onion powder	seasoning
4 tablespoons cornstarch or	1 pound mushrooms,
arrowroot	chopped

Preheat the oven to 350°F.

For the dressing: Place the bread in a bowl. Add the hot water, cover, and set aside. Sauté the onion and celery in the ¾ cup water and cook until soft. Combine all of the dressing ingredients and mix well. Shape the dressing into an oval patty and add bread crumbs or more hot water, if necessary, to attain the desired consistency. Place on a flat nonstick baking sheet with sides. Bake for 1 hour, or until firm and lightly browned. Set aside but don't turn off the oven.

For the vegebird: Grind the warm rice in a food chopper or food processor. Sauté the onion in a small amount of water and add to the cooked ground rice. Mix in the remaining vegebird ingredients. Cover the entire baked dressing with the warm rice mixture and form into a turkey shape. Save enough mixture to make two "drumsticks" and "wings." Attach the "drumsticks" to the turkey with skewer sticks. Form and press the "wings." Baste very lightly with oil and bake at 350°F for 15 minutes. Baste lightly again and bake 20 to 30 minutes more, or until golden brown.

For the gravy: Brown the flour in a dry skillet, stirring, for several minutes. Cool. Then blend the flour, 1 cup of the water, the cashews, onion powder, cornstarch, garlic powder, pepper, and poultry seasoning until smooth, in a blender or food processor.

When creamy, add the remaining 3 cups of water and blend. Pour into a saucepan and cook over medium heat, stirring constantly, until thick, about 5 minutes. Cook the chopped mushrooms in a small amount of water until soft. Then add to the gravy for "giblets."

SPECIAL SEASONING

2 tablespoons celery seeds	½ teaspoon garlic powder
2 tablespoons onion powder	¼ teaspoon dried marjoram
2 tablespoons parsley flakes	¼ teaspoon dried savory
2 tablespoons ground turmeric	

Combine all of the ingredients and store in a tightly sealed jar.

Upper-Crust Stuffing

SERVINGS: 8 TO 10
PREPARATION TIME: 1 HOUR, 15 MINUTES
COOKING TIME: 1½ HOURS

10 small potatoes	1 teaspoon dried marjoram
1½ loaves stale whole-wheat bread	1 teaspoon dried thyme
1 onion, chopped	1 teaspoon poultry seasoning
2 stalks celery, chopped	½ teaspoon dried rosemary
3½ cups water	¼ teaspoon freshly ground pepper (optional)
1 tablespoon vegetable bouillon mix	Paprika to taste
1 tablespoon parsley flakes	2 tablespoons soy sauce
2 teaspoons dried sage	

Peel the potatoes and cut them in half. Cook in water to cover until just tender, about 30 minutes. Drain off the water, reserving 1 cup. Mash the potatoes with small amounts of the water, adding more if the potatoes seem too dry. Set aside.

Cube the bread into ½-inch pieces. Place in a large bowl. Set aside.

Place the onion and celery in a saucepan with ½ cup of the water. Cook over medium-high heat until the onion is translucent, stirring frequently. Add the remaining 3 cups water, the bouillon mix, all seasonings except the paprika, and soy sauce. Cover and cook over medium heat for 15 minutes.

Add the liquid to the bread and mix well. Cover and let rest for 15 minutes.

Preheat the oven to 350°F.

Place the bread mixture in a large casserole dish. Cover with the mashed potatoes. Sprinkle with the paprika and more pepper to taste. Bake for 1 hour, or until the potatoes are golden.

Savory Loaf

SERVINGS: 6 TO 8
PREPARATION TIME: 15 MINUTES (NEED COOKED RICE)
COOKING TIME: 1 HOUR

This also makes a great stuffing. Or serve it as a "sloppy Joe," covered with marinara sauce.

- 1 cup low-fat soy milk or rice milk (see Note)
- 3 teaspoons Ener-G Egg Replacer
- 1¾ cups cooked short-grain brown rice
- ¼ cup cooked wild rice
- 2 cups whole-wheat bread crumbs
- 1 cup chopped walnuts (optional)
- 1½ cups finely chopped onion
- 1 cup finely chopped celery
- 2 tablespoons chopped fresh parsley (or 1 tablespoon dried)
- 2 tablespoons soy sauce
- 1 teaspoon dried basil
- ¼ teaspoon dried sage
- ¼ teaspoon paprika
- Dash freshly ground black pepper
- ¼ teaspoon salt (optional)

Preheat the oven to 350°F.

Add the Egg Replacer to the soy or rice milk and mix in a blender until foamy.

Place all of the ingredients into a bowl and mix together well. Press firmly into a nonstick loaf pan and bake for 1 hour or until firm.

Slide a thin, sharp knife between the loaf and the pan. Place a serving plate on top and turn over (quickly), letting the loaf drop out onto the plate. Serve with mushroom gravy or another sauce of your choice.

Note: Cashew milk can be used, but it makes for a richer loaf. To make a thick cashew milk, use ½ cup cashews blended with ¾ cup water.

CHAPTER 8

SIDE DISHES

The side dishes in this chapter are different than what you've known because they are not soaked in butter, mayonnaise, or vegetable oil, so you can taste the fresh flavors of the ingredients. These side dishes don't make up the centerpiece of the meal, but they can be an effective way to lose weight by filling your stomach with very low-fat, low-calorie choices. They are also packed full of nutrients.

Familiar side dishes, such as Stuffed Zucchini, Mustard Squash, and Golden Spicy Cauliflower are easy, instant successes. For those more devoted to the kitchen, you'll want to try Harvest Baked Squash, Stuffed Mushroom Caps, and Oriental Steamed Dumplings. You may find many of these so satisfying that you make an entire meal out of a single side dish.

Dolmas

SERVINGS: MAKES ABOUT 48 STUFFED LEAVES
PREPARATION TIME: 45 MINUTES (NEED COOKED RICE)
COOKING TIME: 20 MINUTES

One 8-ounce dry weight jar
    grape leaves
2 small sweet onions,
    finely chopped
2 cloves garlic, crushed
½ cup water
3 cups cooked long-grain
    brown rice
¼ cup finely chopped
    fresh parsley

⅓ cup currants
1 tablespoon fresh lemon
    juice
1 tablespoon soy sauce
¼ teaspoon freshly ground
    pepper (or more to taste)
Lemon wedges for
    garnish

Place the grape leaves in a pan of warm water to separate. Remove and drain on paper towels.

Combine the remaining ingredients, except the lemon wedges, in a bowl.

Place a grape leaf, vein side up, stem toward you, on your work surface. Place a mound of the filling just behind the stem (1 teaspoon to 1 tablespoon, depending on the leaf size). Fold over the sides and roll the leaf tightly. Place it in a large, flat, 12-inch skillet. Repeat until all of the filling mixture is used, placing the rolls in a single layer, side by side.

Carefully pour in 2 cups of water. Weight the *dolmas* with a heavy heatproof plate that fits in the pan. Cover. Bring to a boil, reduce the heat, and simmer for 20 minutes. Serve hot or cold, garnished with lemon wedges.

Potato Kugel

SERVINGS: 6 TO 8
PREPARATION TIME: 45 MINUTES
COOKING TIME: 30 MINUTES

This can be served as is or with a sauce, such as Tangy Mushroom Sauce, Brown Gravy, or Szechwan Sauce.

2 **pounds potatoes, peeled**
   and cut into large chunks
1 **medium onion, finely**
   chopped

¾ **cup water**
Freshly ground pepper to
taste
Paprika to taste

Place the potatoes in a saucepan and cover with cold water. Bring to a boil, cover, and cook over medium heat until tender, about 20 minutes.

Meanwhile, place the onion in a nonstick frying pan with ½ cup water. Cook, stirring, until the water evaporates and the onion begins to stick to the pan. Add another ¼ cup water and repeat the procedure. Remove from the heat and set aside.

When the potatoes are tender, drain and reserve the cooking liquid. Mash the potatoes until smooth, using some of the reserved liquid to moisten. Stir in the onion and freshly ground pepper to taste.

Preheat the oven to 375°F.

Fill a 9-inch square, nonstick pan with the potato mixture. Sprinkle with more freshly ground pepper and paprika. Bake for 30 minutes, or until firm and lightly browned.

Notes: Save the potato cooking liquid and use as a vegetable stock in other recipes. Leftovers may be frozen. Reheat, covered, in the oven at 300°F for about 30 minutes.

Baked Potato Skins

SERVINGS: VARIABLE
PREPARATION TIME: 5 MINUTES
COOKING TIME: 1 HOUR

Serve with an oil-free dressing or salsa.

Medium-size baking potatoes	Seasonings of your choice, optional
	Oil-free dressing, optional

Preheat the oven to 450°F.

Scrub the potatoes and prick them several times with a fork. Bake for 45 to 50 minutes. Cut the potatoes in half lengthwise. Gently scoop out the insides of the potatoes, leaving about ¼ inch next to the skin. Reserve the insides for other uses.

Turn on the broiler. Season the potato skins with the seasonings of your choice or brush them with a small amount of oil-free dressing. Place them on a broiler pan and broil until lightly browned. Watch them carefully to make sure they don't burn.

Golden Potato Wedges

SERVINGS: VARIABLE
PREPARATION TIME: 5 MINUTES
COOKING TIME: 45 TO 60 MINUTES

Serve as is or with catsup, salsa, or barbecue sauce.

Baking potatoes, scrubbed	Seasonings of your choice

Preheat the oven to 400°F.

Cut the potatoes lengthwise into wedges. Sprinkle with some of your favorite salt-free seasoning mix. (Garlic powder and paprika are good choices.) Bake on a nonstick baking sheet for 45 to 60 minutes, or until they are easily pierced with a fork.

Grated Potato Bake

SERVINGS: 4
PREPARATION TIME: 20 MINUTES
COOKING TIME: 45 TO 50 MINUTES

For a lovely breakfast dish, make this with potatoes and onion only.

4 medium potatoes (baking, new, or yellow Finns), peeled and very coarsely grated

2 carrots, scrubbed and very coarsely grated

1 stalk celery, diced

1 medium onion, chopped

2 cloves garlic, finely chopped

1 tablespoon finely chopped fresh parsley or dill

Preheat the oven to 350°F.

Mix all of the ingredients well in a large bowl. Put a little water in the bottom of a 3-quart casserole and spoon in the vegetables. Bake, covered, for 45 to 50 minutes, or until lightly browned.

Scalloped Potatoes with Corn

SERVINGS: 6 TO 8
PREPARATION TIME: 20 MINUTES
COOKING TIME: 1 HOUR, 15 MINUTES

2 pounds potatoes
2 tablespoons whole-wheat flour
White pepper to taste
Paprika to taste
1½ cups frozen corn kernels
2½ cups soy milk

Preheat the oven to 350°F.

Scrub the potatoes or peel them if you wish. Cut them into ⅛-inch-thick slices. Layer one-third of the potatoes into a 2-quart casserole. Sprinkle with half of the flour and the pepper and paprika to taste. Spread half of the corn over this. Repeat with another third of the potatoes, the remaining flour, more of the pepper and paprika, and the remaining corn. Finish with the final third of the potatoes. Pour the soy milk over the vegetables. Cover and bake for 30 minutes. Uncover and bake for another 45 minutes, or until the sauce has thickened slightly and the potatoes are lightly browned on top. Let stand for a few minutes before serving.

Spicy Potato Chunks

SERVINGS: 6 TO 8
PREPARATION TIME: 20 MINUTES
COOKING TIME: 30 TO 45 MINUTES

½ teaspoon paprika
¼ teaspoon cayenne
2 teaspoons dried tarragon
1 teaspoon dry mustard
1 tablespoon Dijon mustard
1 to 2 cloves minced garlic
8 to 9 medium potatoes, scrubbed and cut into 1-inch chunks

Preheat the oven to 425°F.

Mix all of the seasonings in a large bowl until you have a smooth paste.

Add a few potato chunks at a time and coat with the seasoning mixture. Repeat until all of the potato pieces are coated. (The less potato you have, the spicier the chunks will be.) Spread out on two nonstick baking sheets and bake for 30 to 45 minutes, or until tender.

Baked Potato Patties

SERVINGS: 4
PREPARATION TIME: 20 MINUTES
COOKING TIME: 30 MINUTES

6 medium potatoes, scrubbed

2 tablespoons minced onion

1 tablespoon chopped fresh parsley

⅛ teaspoon freshly ground black pepper

2 tablespoons whole-wheat pastry flour

Preheat the oven to 375°F.

Shred the potatoes coarsely. Mix with the onion, parsley, pepper, and flour. Shape into four patties and place on a nonstick baking sheet. Bake for 30 minutes. If you like, place the patties under the broiler during the last few minutes for browning.

Sweet-Potato Puffs

SERVINGS: 6 TO 8
PREPARATION TIME: 20 MINUTES
COOKING TIME: 1 HOUR

¼ cup millet
1¼ cups water
5 medium sweet potatoes, peeled and cubed
1 large clove garlic, minced
1 medium onion, finely chopped
1 small stalk celery with leaves, sliced thinly
1 carrot, scrubbed and grated
¼ teaspoon dried basil

Preheat the oven to 350°F.

Place the millet in a saucepan with ¾ cup of the water. Cook over low heat for 30 to 40 minutes, or until softened. Meanwhile, steam the sweet potatoes until soft, about 15 minutes. Mash them well. Sauté the garlic, onion, celery, and carrot in the remaining ½ cup water until tender, about 7 minutes. Combine the millet, potatoes, vegetables, and basil, and mix well.

Drop the mixture by tablespoons onto a nonstick baking sheet, being careful not to flatten the puffs. Bake for 20 minutes, or until lightly browned.

Seasoned Oven Fries

SERVINGS: 4
PREPARATION TIME: 5 MINUTES
COOKING TIME: 45 MINUTES
MARINATING TIME: 1 HOUR

4 large potatoes   **1 cup oil-free Italian dressing**

Thickly slice the potatoes lengthwise. Place the potatoes in a flat baking dish. Pour the dressing over the potatoes and marinate for 1 hour, turning occasionally to make sure that all are coated with dressing.

Preheat the oven to 450°F.

Place the potatoes on a nonstick baking sheet. Bake for 45 minutes, or until lightly browned, basting occasionally with dressing.

Potato Balls

SERVINGS: 4 TO 5
PREPARATION TIME: 25 MINUTES (NEED COOKED POTATOES)
COOKING TIME: 15 TO 20 MINUTES

4 to 5 potatoes, peeled and boiled until just tender
¼ cup finely chopped onion
1½ teaspoon dried basil

½ teaspoon garlic powder
1 teaspoon brewer's yeast
⅓ cup fine bread crumbs

Preheat the oven to 350°F.

Finely shred the potatoes with a grater or in a food processor. Mix with all of the other ingredients, except the bread crumbs. Roll into little balls (about 1½ inches in diameter). Roll in the bread crumbs. Place on a nonstick baking sheet and bake for 15 to 20 minutes, or until brown. Turn once or twice for even browning.

Baked Harvest Squash

SERVINGS: 8
PREPARATION TIME: 10 TO 25 MINUTES
COOKING TIME: 20 MINUTES

4 small acorn squash
1 large green apple, chopped
½ cup diced water chestnuts
¼ cup water

1 recipe Cranberry Sauce
(page 341)
1 teaspoon ground cinnamon
½ teaspoon grated fresh
ginger

Halve the squash; remove the seeds and stringy portions. Place the squash, cut-sides down, in a microwaveproof baking dish. Cover with waxed paper and microwave on High until tender, about 8 minutes. (If you do not have a microwave oven, place the squash in a large pan with 1 inch of water in the bottom. Cover and steam until tender, about 20 minutes.) When the squash is done, place, cut sides up, in a large baking dish and set aside.

Preheat the oven to 400°F.

Sauté the apple and water chestnuts in the water until tender, about 10 minutes. Add the Cranberry Sauce, cinnamon, and ginger. Mix well and remove from the heat. Spoon into the squash halves. Bake for 10 minutes.

Stuffed Zucchini

SERVINGS: 2 TO 4
PREPARATION TIME: 30 MINUTES
COOKING TIME: 1 HOUR

1 large zucchini (big
enough to stuff)
1 cup finely chopped
onion

1 cup finely chopped
celery
1 to 2 cloves garlic, pressed
⅓ cup water

3 tablespoons chopped
fresh parsley

1 medium tomato,
chopped

1 cup whole-wheat bread
crumbs

Cut the zucchini in half lengthwise. Steam over boiling water for 2 to 3 minutes. Remove from the pan and immediately dunk in cold water. Drain. Scoop out the flesh, leaving only a small amount next to the skin so the halves look like canoes. Chop the zucchini flesh and set aside.

Preheat the oven to 325°F.

Cook the onion, celery, and garlic in the water for 5 minutes. Add the zucchini flesh, parsley, and tomato. Cook for another 5 minutes.

Stuff the mixture into the zucchini "boats" and top with the bread crumbs. Place in a casserole and bake for 30 minutes, covered; uncover and bake for 15 minutes, or until the zucchini is tender and the tops are lightly browned.

Mustard Squash

SERVINGS: 4

PREPARATION TIME: 10 MINUTES   COOKING TIME: 15 MINUTES

3 medium zucchini, sliced

1 medium yellow summer
squash or 4 pattypan
squash, sliced

½ cup vegetable broth (page
132) or water

2 tablespoons white wine

3 scallions, finely chopped

1 tablespoon cornstarch

1½ teaspoons slivered fresh
tarragon or dill

1 teaspoon Dijon mustard

⅛ teaspoon freshly ground
black pepper

Steam the zucchini and summer squash over boiling water for about 10 minutes, or until tender. Remove from the heat, drain, and set aside.

Combine the remaining ingredients in a saucepan. Cook, stirring constantly, over medium heat until the mixture boils and thickens, about 5 minutes. Pour the sauce over the squash mixture; toss gently to mix. Serve at once.

Spiced Rice

SERVINGS: 4
PREPARATION TIME: 10 MINUTES
COOKING TIME: 50 MINUTES, PLUS 15 MINUTES RESTING TIME

¼ cup water	⅛ teaspoon ground ginger
1 medium onion, thinly sliced	Dash cayenne
	Dash ground cinnamon
1 clove garlic, minced	Dash ground cumin
1 cup long-grain brown rice	Dash ground nutmeg
¼ teaspoon ground cardamom	1¼ cups vegetable broth
	½ cup raisins

In a medium saucepan, cook the onion and garlic in the water for 5 minutes, stirring frequently. Stir in the rice and all of the seasonings. Cook, stirring for about 3 minutes, to blend the flavors. Add the vegetable broth. Bring to a boil; reduce the heat. Cover and simmer for 30 minutes. Add the raisins, stir gently, cover, and continue to cook for an additional 15 minutes. Remove from the heat. Let stand, covered, for 15 minutes.

Indian Rice

SERVINGS: 2
PREPARATION TIME: 15 MINUTES   COOKING TIME: 1 HOUR

The person who sent me this recipe wrote, "This is a favorite recipe because it requires no tending. I can prepare it before work, except for the baking, set the oven timer, and have it finished when I return home." Serve with a bean salad or one of the main dish vegetables, such as Potato Curry or Harvest Vegetable Sauté.

1 medium onion, chopped	½ teaspoon curry powder
¼ cup water	2 cups boiling water
½ cup raisins	¼ cup slivered almonds
½ cup long-grain brown rice	(optional)

Preheat the oven to 350°F.

Sauté the onion in the water for about 5 minutes. Add the raisins, rice, and curry. Stir to mix. Add the boiling water. Pour into a 1½-quart casserole dish. Bake, covered, for 50 to 55 minutes. Lightly toast the almonds in a dry nonstick skillet, then stir them in.

Quick Bulghur with Pasta

SERVINGS: 2
PREPARATION TIME: 5 MINUTES
COOKING TIME: 15 MINUTES, PLUS 5 MINUTES RESTING TIME

Serve this instead of cooked brown rice for a delicious variation.

2 cups water	¼ teaspoon dried basil
1 cup bulghur	¼ teaspoon dried oregano
⅓ cup small pasta (orzo, small shells, small bows, or alphabets)	

Bring the water to a boil in a small saucepan. Add the remaining ingredients. Reduce the heat to low. Cover the pan and cook for 15 minutes. Remove from the heat. Fluff with a fork and let stand for 5 minutes before serving.

Oats and Millet

SERVINGS: 2
PREPARATION TIME: 10 MINUTES
COOKING TIME: 30 TO 35 MINUTES

Use this recipe as you would cooked brown rice. Delicious with any of your favorite sauces. Try Broccoli Cheese Sauce or Tangy Mushroom Sauce.

½ cup millet
2 cups water
½ cup steel-cut oats
½ teaspoon salt

Fresh or dried herbs to taste (oregano, basil, tarragon, dill, chervil)

Place the millet in a large cast-iron skillet over medium heat and toast for 5 to 10 minutes, stirring frequently to prevent scorching. Bring the water to a boil in a saucepan. Add the remaining ingredients, including the toasted millet. Cover the pan and cook over low heat for 30 to 35 minutes. Stir before serving.

Three-Grain Medley

SERVINGS: 2
PREPARATION TIME: 5 MINUTES
COOKING TIME: 45 MINUTES

Use this instead of cooked brown rice for a delicious variation. Serve with your favorite sauces.

1¾ cups water
⅓ cup long-grain brown rice

⅓ cup whole oat groats
⅓ cup barley

Bring the water to a boil. Add the remaining ingredients. Cover and cook over low heat for 45 minutes.

Five-Grain Medley

SERVINGS: VARIABLE (1 CUP OF THE RICE MIXTURE WILL YIELD
ABOUT 3 CUPS COOKED)
PREPARATION TIME: 5 MINUTES
COOKING TIME: 1 HOUR, PLUS OPTIONAL 15 MINUTES RESTING TIME

Try this healthful grain mixture topped with your favorite sauces.

2 cups long-grain
brown rice
¼ cup barley

¼ cup millet
¼ cup rye berries
¼ cup wheat berries

Mix the grains in a bowl. Store in a tightly covered jar until ready
to use.

To cook, place 1 cup of the grain mixture in a saucepan. Add
2½ cups of water and bring to a boil. Reduce the heat, cover, and
cook over low heat until the water is absorbed, 45 to 60 minutes.
For fluffier grains, let the mixture rest for 15 minutes before stirring
and serving.

Barbecued Onions

SERVINGS: VARIABLE
PREPARATION TIME: 5 MINUTES
COOKING TIME: 20 MINUTES

Serve as a garnish on burgers, sandwiches, potatoes, or whatever sounds good to you.

We also like these without the barbecue sauce—just cooked, browned onions.

2 large onions, chopped   **¼ cup barbecue sauce of**
1½ to 2 cups water   **your choice**

Place the onions in a large nonstick frying pan with 1 cup of the water. Cook over medium heat, stirring occasionally, until the liquid evaporates and the onions begin to stick to the bottom of the pan, about 10 minutes. Add another ¼ cup water and continue to cook, stirring, until the water evaporates and the onions again begin to stick. Repeat this one or two more times, until the onions are very soft and brown. Mix in the barbecue sauce.

Stuffed Mushroom Caps

SERVINGS: 12
PREPARATION TIME: 30 MINUTES
COOKING TIME: 25 MINUTES

These can also be served as a hot appetizer.

22 to 24 extra-large
   mushrooms, or 38 to
   40 medium-large
   mushrooms
¼ cup water
1 large onion, finely
   chopped
2 cloves garlic, pressed

2 cups packed, chopped
   fresh spinach
1 tablespoon soy sauce
¾ cup Bread Crumb
   Mixture
   (page 128)
   Freshly ground
   pepper to taste

Preheat the oven to 350°F.

Clean the mushrooms, remove the stems, and set them aside. Place the mushroom caps, stem-side up, on a nonstick baking sheet. Chop the mushroom stems finely.

Place the water, onion, and garlic in a large nonstick frying pan. Cook, stirring for 2 minutes. Add the mushroom stems and cook for 2 more minutes. Add the spinach and soy sauce. Cook for another 2 minutes or so, until the spinach is wilted. Stir in the bread crumbs. Cook over low heat until all of the moisture is absorbed. Season with pepper.

Place a small amount of the spinach mixture in each mushroom cap. Repeat until all are filled. Cover with parchment paper, then cover with foil, turning the edges under to seal. Bake for 15 minutes, or until the mushrooms are just tender.

Brussels Sprouts with Creamy Horseradish Sauce

SERVINGS: 4
PREPARATION TIME: 15 MINUTES
COOKING TIME: 10 TO 15 MINUTES

Try the sauce over baked potatoes or other steamed vegetables.

1 pound fresh Brussels
sprouts
½ cup Herb Magic
Creamy Cucumber
Dressing (see Note)

½ to 1 teaspoon prepared
horseradish (oil- and
dairy-free)

Wash the Brussels sprouts thoroughly and remove any discolored leaves. Trim off the stem ends. Steam over boiling water for 10 to 15 minutes, until just tender. Drain. Place in a bowl and cover.

Combine the dressing with the horseradish, using more or less of the latter, according to taste. Pour over the Brussels sprouts; serve.

Note: Creamy Cucumber Dressing is oil- and dairy-free.

Green Bean Medley

SERVINGS: 4 TO 6
PREPARATION TIME: 20 MINUTES
COOKING TIME: 30 MINUTES

1 medium onion, chopped
½ pound mushrooms,
chopped
1 medium red bell pepper,
chopped
2 cloves garlic, minced

1 cup water
3 tablespoons soy sauce
1 pound green beans,
trimmed and cut into
1½-inch pieces

Place the onion, mushrooms, bell pepper, and garlic in a nonstick frying pan with ½ cup of the water. Cook, stirring frequently, until the water evaporates and the vegetables begin to stick to the bottom of the pan. Add ¼ cup of the remaining water. Cook, stirring, until the water evaporates and the vegetables begin to stick. Add the remaining water and repeat this step. Add the soy sauce, mix well, and set aside.

Steam the green beans over boiling water until tender, 10 to 15 minutes. Remove from the heat and place in a bowl. Add the vegetable mixture to the beans; toss to mix and serve at once.

Golden Spicy Cauliflower

SERVINGS: 4 TO 6
PREPARATION TIME: 15 MINUTES
COOKING TIME: 20 MINUTES

1 medium cauliflower, cut into florets	1 bunch scallions, chopped
2 cloves garlic, pressed	2 tablespoons rice vinegar
2 to 3 tablespoons grated fresh ginger	2 tablespoons soy sauce
1 cup water	½ teaspoon ground turmeric
2 medium tomatoes, seeded and chopped	Freshly ground pepper to taste

Place the cauliflower, garlic, and ginger in a saucepan with ½ cup of the water. Cook, stirring occasionally, for about 10 minutes. Add the remaining water and the rest of the ingredients. Bring to a boil, reduce the heat, and simmer, covered, until the cauliflower is tender, about 10 minutes longer. Stir occasionally during cooking to prevent the cauliflower from sticking to the bottom of the pan.

Sautéed Italian Zucchini

SERVINGS: 4
PREPARATION TIME: 10 MINUTES
COOKING TIME: 10 MINUTES

¼ cup water
1 clove garlic, minced
5 to 6 small zucchini (1 pound), trimmed and sliced

2 tablespoons soy sauce
2 tablespoons chopped fresh parsley
½ teaspoon dried oregano
½ teaspoon dried basil

Put the water and garlic in a pan. Add the remaining ingredients. Sauté, stirring occasionally, until softened but not mushy, about 10 minutes.

Dutch Vegetable Whip

SERVINGS: 4
PREPARATION TIME: 20 MINUTES
COOKING TIME: 30 MINUTES

3 cups peeled and diced potato
1 cup scrubbed and diced carrot
½ onion, sliced

1 teaspoon chopped fresh parsley
⅛ teaspoon freshly ground pepper
¾ cup water

Place all of the ingredients in a saucepan. Cover and cook over medium heat until tender, about 30 minutes. Mash with a potato masher or electric beater.

Variations: 1. Add 1 peeled and chopped tart apple to the ingredients. Cook and mash as above.
2. Substitute 1 cup chopped cabbage or escarole for the carrot.

Dutch Red Cabbage

SERVINGS: 8
PREPARATION TIME: 15 MINUTES
COOKING TIME: 1 HOUR

1 small head red cabbage, thinly sliced
1 to 2 tart apples, chopped
¼ cup cider vinegar

1 cup sugar-free raspberry jam
¼ cup water

Place all of the ingredients in a saucepan. Cover and simmer over low heat until the cabbage is tender, about 1 hour, stirring occasionally.

Jiffy Vegetarian Posole

SERVINGS: 6
PREPARATION TIME: 5 MINUTES
COOKING TIME: 15 MINUTES

Serve as an appetizer or side dish with a Mexican dinner.

Two 15-ounce cans hominy
½ to 1 teaspoon chili powder

½ teaspoon cumin seeds, crushed (see Note)

Combine all of the ingredients in a saucepan. Simmer over low heat for 15 minutes.

Note: Crush the seeds with a mortar and pestle or put them into a small plastic bag and gently smash with a hammer.

Gingered Carrots

SERVINGS: 4 TO 6
PREPARATION TIME: 10 MINUTES
COOKING TIME: 15 MINUTES

6 large carrots, scrubbed
and sliced
One ½-inch piece fresh
ginger, grated (1
tablespoon)

Grated zest of ½ orange
1 tablespoon honey
Fresh parsley sprigs for
garnish

Cook the carrots in ½ inch of water, covered, until tender, about
15 minutes. Add the ginger, orange zest, and honey. Stir well. Serve
hot, garnished with fresh parsley sprigs.

Oriental Steamed Dumplings

SERVINGS: MAKES ABOUT 30 TO 40 DUMPLINGS
PREPARATION TIME: 1 HOUR
COOKING TIME: 10 MINUTES PER BATCH

*My daughter likes to eat these cold, so I always make plenty to be sure she
has leftovers for a few days afterwards. Serve with soy sauce and hot mustard.*

½ pound mushrooms,
finely chopped
1 bunch scallions,
finely chopped
1½ cups shredded bok
choy
4 cups shredded Napa
cabbage
½ cup water
2 cups bean sprouts
½ pound firm tofu,
cut into 1½ × ¼-
inch strips

3 tablespoons soy sauce
⅛ teaspoon sesame oil
(optional)
½ teaspoon ground
ginger or 1 teaspoon
grated fresh ginger
2 tablespoons
cornstarch, mixed
with 2 tablespoons
cold water
30 to 40 egg-roll wrappers

In a wok or a large frying pan, sauté the mushrooms, onion, bok coy, and cabbage in the ½ cup water for 5 minutes. Add the sprouts, tofu, soy sauce, sesame oil, and ginger. Simmer for 10 minutes. Add the cornstarch mixture. Cook, stirring, until thickened. Set aside and let cool.

Place one eggroll wrapper on the counter like a diamond. (Cover the remaining wrappers with a damp cloth to prevent them from drying out.) Take about 1 heaping tablespoon of filling and squeeze out the excess liquid. Spread the filling on the lower third of the wrapper. Starting at the point closest to you, bring the bottom half of the wrapper up to enclose the filling. Fold in the two sides and continue rolling up the dumpling. Brush a little water over the inside of the tip and press the edges together.

Line a steamer basket with parchment paper or lettuce or cabbage leaves to keep the dumplings from sticking. Set the filled dumplings in the basket over boiling water. Cover and steam for 10 minutes, or until the wrappers are translucent.

CHAPTER 9

SAUCES

The foundation of a meal, whether it is poultry or potatoes, has little taste but has great influence on your health because it provides the bulk of the food intake. The accompanying sauce, however, provides almost all of the enjoyment of the meal, as sauces contain delightful combinations of spices and arrays of colorful vegetables.

How adventuresome are you? Some of the more intriguing sauces in this section are Cajun Vegetable Sauce, Turkeyless à la King Sauce, Mideast Vegetable Sauce, Yellow Pepper Sauce, Fresh Tomato and Garlic Sauce.

When planning a meal, decide on a sauce, then choose the starch that will form the base of your meal. Try some different combinations. There is nothing sacred about always using pasta with spaghetti sauce; try it over potatoes or spaghetti squash. Other great combinations are Shiitaki Mushroom Sauce over potatoes, Cranberry Sauce over sweet potatoes, and Red Pepper Sauce as a dip for fresh sourdough bread. These are just a few possibilities—the variations are limitless.

Simple Sauces

Tangy Mushroom Sauce

SERVINGS: MAKES 2 CUPS
PREPARATION TIME: 10 MINUTES
COOKING TIME: 25 MINUTES

Serve over potatoes or whole grains.

¼ pound mushrooms (8 large), sliced
1 leek, washed and sliced
2 cups water
1 tablespoon soy sauce
1 teaspoon parsley flakes

¼ teaspoon dried oregano
¼ teaspoon dried sage
⅛ teaspoon paprika
Freshly ground white pepper
2 tablespoons cornstarch

Sauté the mushrooms and leek in ½ cup of the water for 5 minutes. Add an additional 1 cup of water and all the seasonings. Cook over low heat for 15 minutes. Mix the cornstarch in the remaining ½ cup cold water. Slowly add to the sauce while stirring. Cook, stirring, until thickened and clear.

Garlic-Mushroom Sauce

SERVINGS: MAKES 2 CUPS
PREPARATION TIME: 10 MINUTES   COOKING TIME: 6 MINUTES

Try this with mixed grain dishes or soba noodles.

1 cup sliced mushrooms
1¾ cups water
2 tablespoons soy sauce
1 clove garlic, pressed
1 teaspoon grated fresh
  ginger

2½ tablespoons cornstarch,
  dissolved in ¼ cup water
Freshly ground pepper to
  taste
Dash sesame oil

Place the mushrooms in a saucepan with ¼ cup of the water. Add the soy sauce, garlic, and ginger. Sauté until the mushrooms are softened slightly, about 4 minutes. Add the remaining 1½ cups water and the cornstarch mixture. Cook, stirring until the mixture boils and thickens. Season with the pepper and sesame oil.

Savory Mushroom Gravy

SERVINGS: MAKES 1 QUART
PREPARATION TIME: 15 MINUTES
COOKING TIME: 30 MINUTES

Delicious over Savory Loaf or over baked or mashed potatoes, as well as over rice.

1¾ cups vegetable broth
  (page 132) or water
4 tablespoons barley
  miso (red or
  traditional)
1 onion, chopped
2 cups sliced mushrooms
  (about ½ pound)

2 to 3 teaspoons dried sage (to
  taste)
2 teaspoons dried thyme
4 tablespoons arrowroot,
  dissolved in ¼ cup
  water
Dash freshly ground
  pepper

Bring the broth or water to a boil. Spoon the miso into the boiling liquid and stir to dissolve. Add the onion, mushrooms, sage, and thyme. Simmer for 15 to 20 minutes, stirring occasionally. Add the dissolved arrowroot to the mixture. Stir until thickened, about 5 minutes. Add a dash of fresh pepper and more miso if a stronger gravy taste is desired.

Mushroom-Garlic Cream Sauce

SERVINGS: MAKES ABOUT 2 CUPS
PREPARATION TIME: 20 MINUTES
COOKING TIME: 25 MINUTES

Serve over brown rice, mashed potatoes, whole-wheat toast, bread stuffing, or any other starch.

12 cloves garlic, peeled
1½ cups water
5 mushrooms, cut in half
Pinch ground nutmeg

¼ cup powdered soy milk (Ener-G Pure Soy Quick)
1 tablespoon cornstarch, mixed with 2 tablespoons cold water

Blanch the garlic cloves in unsalted boiling water three times, changing the water each time.

Combine the 1½ cups water, blanched garlic, mushrooms, and nutmeg in a saucepan. Simmer for 15 minutes over low heat. Stir in the powdered soy milk and simmer for another 5 minutes. Puree in a blender or food processor and return to the pan. Add the cornstarch mixture. Stir continuously until thickened.

Brown Gravy

SERVINGS: MAKES 2 CUPS
PREPARATION TIME: 10 MINUTES   COOKING TIME: 5 MINUTES

Serve over potatoes, steamed vegetables, or grains.

2 cups warm water
1 tablespoon raw cashew
  pieces, rinsed
1 tablespoon onion
  powder
2 tablespoons cornstarch
  or arrowroot
3 tablespoons soy sauce

2 to 3 cloves garlic, pressed,
  or ½ teaspoon garlic
  powder
⅛ teaspoon freshly
  ground black pepper
1 to 2 tablespoons parsley
  flakes (optional)

pinch thyme   pinch of dried mushrooms

Place ½ cup warm water and all of the ingredients except the parsley in a blender or food processor and blend until smooth and creamy.

When creamy, add 1½ cups more warm water and blend. Pour into a saucepan and cook over medium heat, stirring constantly, until thick, about 5 minutes. Add the parsley flakes for color after cooking, if desired.

Garlic Sauce

SERVINGS: 2 LARGE
PREPARATION TIME: 10 MINUTES   COOKING TIME: 10 MINUTES

Serve over pasta.

6 to 8 cloves garlic, thinly
  sliced
1 onion, sliced
One 8.45-ounce package
  low-fat plain soy
  milk

1 heaping tablespoon
  cornstarch
1 heaping tablespoon
  brewer's yeast
Garlic powder to taste
  (optional)

Sauté the garlic and onion in a small amount of water for 3 to 5 minutes. In another pot, mix the soy milk, cornstarch, and yeast. Add the garlic, onion, and any water remaining in the sauté pan. Bring to a boil and cook, stirring constantly, until thickened. For a stronger garlic flavor, add garlic powder to taste.

Fresh Tomato Sauce

SERVINGS: MAKES ABOUT 6 CUPS
PREPARATION TIME: 20 MINUTES
COOKING TIME: 40 MINUTES

Serve over pasta, gnocchi, or spaghetti squash.

4 pounds tomatoes,
  coarsely chopped
1 large onion, chopped
2 to 3 cloves garlic, minced
1 tablespoon chopped
  fresh oregano
1 tablespoon chopped
  fresh thyme

1 bay leaf
¼ teaspoon crushed red
  pepper flakes
¼ cup chopped fresh basil
  Freshly ground pepper
  to taste

Place the tomatoes, onion, garlic, oregano, thyme, bay leaf, and pepper in a large saucepan. Bring to a boil, reduce the heat, and simmer, uncovered, for 30 minutes, stirring occasionally. Remove the bay leaf. Stir in the fresh basil and pepper.

Green Chili Sauce

SERVINGS: MAKES ABOUT 3 QUARTS
PREPARATION TIME: 10 MINUTES
COOKING TIME: 6 TO 8 HOURS

Use this spicy sauce over burritos or rice. It is very hot! (For a milder sauce, use less jalapeño pepper.) You can also prepare this sauce in a slow cooker. It will become thicker and more flavorful the longer it cooks. It also freezes well.

3½ cups water
Four 16-ounce cans whole tomatoes, chopped
Three 15-ounce cans tomato sauce
Four 7-ounce cans chopped green chilies

2 tablespoons diced jalapeño pepper
6 cloves garlic (or 2 tablespoons garlic powder)

Place all of the ingredients in a large pot and simmer for 6 to 8 hours, or as long as possible.

Enchilada Sauce

SERVINGS: MAKES 2½ CUPS
PREPARATION TIME: 10 MINUTES
COOKING TIME: 25 MINUTES

Serve with Bean Burritos.

One 8-ounce can tomato sauce
1½ cups water
1 large onion, chopped
2 cloves garlic, minced
1 tablespoon chili powder

½ teaspoon ground cumin
½ teaspoon dried oregano
2 tablespoons cornstarch, mixed with ¼ cup cold water

Place all of the ingredients except the cornstarch mixture in a small saucepan. Bring to a boil, reduce the heat, cover, and simmer for 20 minutes. Add the cornstarch mixture. Cook, stirring, until thickened.

Chunky Enchilada Sauce

SERVINGS: MAKES ABOUT 6 CUPS
PREPARATION TIME: 15 MINUTES
COOKING TIME: 30 MINUTES

Use this sauce to make bean or vegetable enchiladas. Use as a topping for Mexican-style rice or potato dishes.

1 onion, chopped
2 cloves garlic, crushed
¼ cup water
One 28-ounce can crushed tomatoes
One 4-ounce can chopped green chilies
3 tablespoons chili powder
½ teaspoon ground cumin
1½ cups water
1 tablespoon soy sauce
3 tablespoons cornstarch

Place the onion, garlic, and water in a large saucepan. Cook, stirring, for 5 minutes, until the onion softens slightly. Add the tomatoes, chilies, and the spices. Stir. Cover and cook over low heat for 15 minutes. Add 1 cup of the water and the soy sauce. Mix the cornstarch in the remaining ½ cup water. Add to the sauce while stirring. Cook, stirring, until thickened.

Green Enchilada Sauce

SERVINGS: MAKES 1 QUART
PREPARATION TIME: 5 MINUTES
COOKING TIME: 10 MINUTES

Serve this spicy sauce with bean burritos.

One 7-ounce can Mexican
    green sauce
3½ cups water

4 tablespoons cornstarch
Chopped fresh cilantro
    for garnish (optional)

Combine all of the ingredients except the cilantro. Cook over medium heat, stirring constantly, until the mixture boils and thickens. Add the cilantro just before using.

Tasty Blender Salsa

SERVINGS: MAKES ABOUT 2 CUPS
PREPARATION TIME: 10 MINUTES

Serve with Oven-Baked Tortilla Chips or on burritos, tostadas, etc.

One 15- to 16-ounce can
    whole tomatoes
2 cloves garlic

¼ cup fresh cilantro leaves
1 fresh jalapeño pepper,
    seeded, stem removed

Place all of the ingredients in a blender or food processor. Process until smooth.

Fresh Salsa

SERVINGS: MAKES 2 CUPS
PREPARATION TIME: 15 MINUTES

Use as a topping for burritos or other Mexican-style food, or serve as a dip for Oven-Baked Tortilla Chips or raw vegetables.

2 cups finely chopped tomatoes

1 small onion, finely chopped

⅓ cup chopped canned green chilies

¼ to ⅓ cup finely chopped fresh cilantro

1 tablespoon fresh lime juice

Pinch or two cayenne (optional)

Combine all of the ingredients, except the cayenne, in a small bowl and mix well. Taste. Add the cayenne if your taste buds permit.

Note: This will keep in the refrigerator for about 1 week.

Golden Carrot Sauce

SERVINGS: MAKES 1½ CUPS
PREPARATION TIME: 10 MINUTES
COOKING TIME: 10 MINUTES

Delicious as a topping for Slow-Cooked English Plum Pudding.

3 tablespoons whole-wheat
pastry flour
¼ teaspoon salt (optional)
½ cup honey
⅔ cup boiling water
⅓ cup brandy (or 1 teaspoon
brandy extract)

¼ cup minced carrot
2 tablespoons fresh-
squeezed orange juice
2 tablespoons fresh lemon
juice
Dash ground nutmeg

In small saucepan, combine the flour and salt. Dissolve the honey in the boiling water and add the brandy. (If extract is used, add it last and use ⅓ cup more water.) Add the hot liquid mixture slowly to the flour mixture. Cook over medium heat for 5 minutes, or until thick and clear, stirring constantly. Add the carrot, orange and lemon juices, and the nutmeg. Simmer for 5 minutes longer.

Cilantro Chutney

SERVINGS: MAKES 1½ CUPS
PREPARATION TIME: 10 MINUTES

Serve as a seasoning addition to many different foods. If you like cilantro, you will find many uses for this chutney. It keeps well in a tightly covered jar in the refrigerator.

4 bunches fresh cilantro
3 cloves garlic, peeled
3 to 4 tablespoons fresh
lemon juice

2 tablespoons honey
1 to 2 tablespoons natural
peanut butter

Wash the cilantro well and remove any yellowed leaves and tough stems. Place in a food processor with the garlic. Process until finely chopped. Combine the lemon juice, honey, and peanut butter in a bowl. Combine the two mixtures and mix well.

Tahini Sauce

SERVINGS: MAKES 2 CUPS
PREPARATION TIME: 5 MINUTES

This is a very rich, high-fat sauce. Use sparingly and only as a special treat if you are thin and in good health. Serve with Falafel.

1 cup tahini	**¼ cup fresh lemon juice**
¾ cup water	**1 tablespoon soy sauce**

Combine all of the ingredients in a blender or food processor and blend until smooth. Refrigerate until ready to use.

Cranberry Sauce

SERVINGS: MAKES 1 QUART
PREPARATION TIME: 10 MINUTES   COOKING TIME: 10 MINUTES

Use as a side dish for holiday meals or use in Harvest Baked Squash.

1 pound fresh cranberries, rinsed	**¼ to ½ cup honey**
1 cup fresh-squeezed orange juice	**Grated zest of 1 orange**

Place all of the ingredients in a saucepan. Cover and cook until the cranberries pop, stirring occasionally. The mixture will be slightly thick.

Szechwan Sauce

SERVINGS: MAKES 1½ CUPS
PREPARATION TIME: 10 MINUTES
COOKING TIME: 5 TO 10 MINUTES

Serve over potatoes or grains.

1½ cups water
5 to 6 scallions, chopped
2 tablespoons soy sauce
1½ tablespoons cornstarch
2½ teaspoons grated fresh
  ginger

1 clove garlic, crushed
⅛ teaspoon crushed red
  pepper flakes
Pinch or two cayenne

Combine all of the ingredients in a saucepan. Cook, stirring, over medium heat until the mixture boils and thickens, 5 to 10 minutes.

Super Soy Sauce

SERVINGS: MAKES 1 CUP
PREPARATION TIME: 5 MINUTES

Use as you would plain soy sauce. This adds a wonderful rich flavor to soups, sauces, and salad dressings. Add more water to make a soup stock.

½ cup water
1½ teaspoons fresh lemon
  juice
½ teaspoon vegetable-
  seasoned salt substitute

½ teaspoon dried basil
½ cup brewer's yeast
2 cloves garlic, pressed
3 tablespoons soy sauce

Liquify all of the ingredients in a blender or food processor.

Hearty Sauces

Shiitake Mushroom Sauce

SERVINGS: 6
PREPARATION TIME: 20 MINUTES
COOKING TIME: 15 MINUTES

Serve over brown rice or Five-Grain Medley.

4 cups water
3 ounces dried shiitake or
   oyster mushrooms
1 medium onion, chopped
1 bunch scallions, chopped
2 cloves garlic, minced

1½ tablespoons grated fresh
   ginger
⅓ cup soy sauce
¼ cup sherry or rice vinegar
⅓ cup cornstarch, mixed
   with ½ cup cold water

Boil 2 cups of the water and pour over the dried mushrooms in a bowl. Soak for 15 minutes while you are chopping the vegetables. Remove the mushrooms from the water and squeeze to remove excess water. Strain the water and reserve 1 cup. Set aside.

Cut the tough stems off the mushrooms and discard. Chop the mushrooms into bite-sized pieces. Set aside.

Put the 1 cup of reserved mushroom liquid into a saucepan. Add the chopped onion. Cook, stirring occasionally, until the onion softens, 2 to 3 minutes. Add the scallions, garlic, ginger, soy sauce, sherry or rice vinegar, and the chopped mushrooms. Mix well and add the remaining 2 cups of water. Heat to boiling, stirring occasionally. Add the cornstarch mixture and cook, stirring continually, until thickened and clear.

Eggplant-Mushroom Sauce

SERVINGS: 6 TO 8
PREPARATION TIME: 20 MINUTES
COOKING TIME: 30 MINUTES

Serve over Savory Baked Polenta or whole grains.

1 medium onion, chopped
1 medium eggplant, chopped
½ pound mushrooms, sliced
1 green bell pepper, chopped
2 cloves garlic, minced
½ cup water
One 15-ounce can tomato sauce

One 6-ounce can tomato paste
One 4-ounce jar chopped pimientos, drained
1 tablespoon soy sauce
½ teaspoon dried basil
½ teaspoon dried oregano
Freshly ground pepper to taste

Place the onion, eggplant, mushrooms, green pepper, and garlic in a large pan with the water. Cook, stirring occasionally, over medium-low heat for 10 minutes. Add the remaining ingredients and cook over low heat for 20 minutes.

Cajun Vegetable Sauce

SERVINGS: 6

PREPARATION TIME: 20 MINUTES   COOKING TIME: 22 MINUTES

Serve over pasta, whole grains, or potatoes.

½ cup water
1 onion, coarsely chopped
½ pound mushrooms, sliced
2 cups broccoli florets
2 small zucchini, sliced
1 small yellow crookneck squash, sliced
Two 15-ounce cans stewed tomatoes (see Note)

One 15-ounce can chunky tomato sauce
¼ cup chopped fresh parsley
2 teaspoons finely chopped fresh basil
½ teaspoon Cajun Spices (see below)
½ teaspoon Louisiana hot sauce or Tabasco

Place the water, onion, and mushrooms in a large wok or pot. Cook over medium heat for 3 minutes, stirring frequently. Add the broccoli and continue to cook, stirring, for 2 minutes. Add the zucchini and squash; cook, stirring, for 2 more minutes. Add the remaining ingredients. Cover and cook over low heat for 15 minutes.

Note: Try using the new Cajun-style stewed tomatoes instead of plain tomatoes.

CAJUN SPICES

SERVINGS: MAKES ½ CUP

3 tablespoons paprika
2 teaspoons onion powder
2 teaspoons freshly ground black pepper
2 teaspoons freshly ground white pepper

2 teaspoons cayenne
1 teaspoon dried oregano
1 teaspoon dried thyme
½ teaspoon celery seed

Mix all of the ingredients and store in a tightly covered container.

Red Pepper Sauce

SERVINGS: MAKES 1 CUP
PREPARATION TIME: 10 MINUTES
COOKING TIME: 20 MINUTES

This makes an excellent spread for bread, or a dip for raw vegetables. You can also double the recipe and use it as a pasta sauce.

2 large red bell peppers,
　chopped
1 small onion, chopped
2 cloves garlic, minced
¼ cup water
1½ teaspoons white-wine
　vinegar

⅛ teaspoon crushed red
　pepper flakes
⅛ teaspoon white pepper
　Dash or two Tabasco
½ to 1 tablespoon horseradish
　(optional)

Place the bell peppers, onion, and garlic in a saucepan with the water. Cover and cook over low heat until the peppers are very soft, about 15 minutes. Transfer to a food processor or blender and process until smooth. Return to the saucepan. Add the remaining ingredients. Cook over low heat for 5 minutes, stirring occasionally, to allow the flavors to blend.

Turkeyless à la King Sauce

SERVINGS: 4
PREPARATION TIME: 20 MINUTES
COOKING TIME: 30 MINUTES

Serve over whole-grain toast, rice, baked potatoes, or pasta.

1 onion, chopped
1 green bell pepper, chopped
½ pound mushrooms, sliced
1 stalk celery, sliced
6 to 8 ears canned baby corn, cut in half
1 cup frozen green peas
1 cup water
½ cup whole-wheat flour
3 cups soy or rice milk
One 4-ounce jar chopped pimientos, drained
1 to 2 teaspoons slivered fresh basil
⅛ teaspoon white pepper
2 tablespoons low-sodium soy sauce
1 tablespoon Worcestershire sauce
2 tablespoons cornstarch or arrowroot, mixed with ¼ cup cold water

In a large pan, cook the onion, green pepper, mushrooms, celery, baby corn, and peas in the water for 10 minutes. Stir in the flour and continue to cook for a few minutes, stirring constantly. Slowly add the milk, while stirring. Cook, stirring frequently, until the mixture boils.

Stir in the pimientos. Add the basil, pepper, soy sauce, and Worcestershire sauce. Gradually add the cornstarch mixture to the pan while stirring. Cook, stirring, until the mixture boils and thickens.

Mideast Vegetable Sauce

SERVINGS: 6 TO 8
PREPARATION TIME: 40 MINUTES
COOKING TIME: 35 MINUTES

Serve over brown rice, couscous, bulghur, or another grain.

1 large onion, sliced and separated into rings
4 cloves garlic, minced
¼ cup water
One 28-ounce can whole tomatoes, chopped, with liquid
2 carrots, scrubbed and thickly sliced
2 stalks celery, thickly sliced
5 sweet potatoes, peeled and chunked
2 teaspoons honey
1 teaspoon ground cinnamon
½ teaspoon ground cumin

½ teaspoon freshly ground black pepper
¼ teaspoon ground turmeric
Several dashes cayenne
A few strands saffron (optional)
3 cups broccoli florets
3 cups cauliflower florets
1 red bell pepper, chopped
One 15-ounce can garbanzo beans, drained and rinsed
½ cup raisins
¼ cup chopped scallion for garnish

Place the onion and garlic in a large pot with the water. Cook, stirring, until the onion is soft, about 5 minutes. Add the tomatoes and their liquid, the carrot, celery, sweet potato, and the seasonings. Cover and simmer for 10 minutes. Add the broccoli, cauliflower, and red pepper. Continue to cook for another 10 minutes. Stir in the garbanzos and raisins and cook for another 10 minutes. Ladle over your grain of choice and garnish with the scallion.

Variation: Substitute other vegetables, such as zucchini, green beans, or cabbage, for the broccoli and cauliflower.

Yellow Pepper Sauce

SERVINGS: 6 TO 8
PREPARATION TIME: 20 MINUTES
COOKING TIME: 35 MINUTES

Serve over spinach pasta—the color contrast is wonderful!

4 medium yellow bell peppers
2 medium potatoes
1 cup water
2 tablespoons white wine

1 tablespoon fresh lemon juice
1½ teaspoons soy sauce
1 teaspoon onion powder
¼ teaspoon freshly ground white pepper

Clean and chop the peppers and peel and chop the potatoes. Place in a saucepan with the water. Cover and cook over low heat for 30 minutes. Remove from the heat. Pour into a blender or food processor. Blend until smooth. Return to the saucepan and add the remaining ingredients. Heat through to allow the flavors to blend.

Mama Lucia Marinara Sauce

SERVINGS: MAKES ABOUT 6 CUPS
PREPARATION TIME: 15 MINUTES
COOKING TIME: 40 MINUTES

*We got this recipe from a family in Hawaii. It has been around for years,
handed down from a woman known as Mama Lucia.*
Serve over your favorite pasta.

1 small onion, chopped
½ pound mushrooms, sliced
¼ cup sherry or white wine
One 15-ounce can water-packed artichoke hearts, drained
One 28-ounce can whole tomatoes, chopped, with liquid

One 15-ounce can tomato sauce
1 bay leaf
½ teaspoon Italian herbs
½ teaspoon dried oregano
¼ teaspoon dried basil

Sauté the onion and mushrooms in the sherry or wine for 5 minutes. Add the artichoke hearts and cook for another 5 minutes. Add the remaining ingredients, cover, and simmer for 30 minutes.

Variation: The person who sent me this recipe likes to add about 12 to 14 sliced green olives to the sauce along with the artichokes. They add an interesting flavor to the sauce but also a significant amount of fat, so consider this an optional step.

Fresh Tomato and Garlic Sauce

SERVINGS: MAKES ABOUT 1 QUART
PREPARATION TIME: 30 MINUTES
COOKING TIME: 10 MINUTES

This is a fresh-tasting garlicky sauce that goes well with any pasta.

6 to 8 large ripe tomatoes
(about 4 to 4½ pounds)
6 to 8 cloves garlic
2 to 3 tablespoons soy sauce
¼ teaspoon crushed red
pepper flakes
Freshly ground pepper
to taste

1 to 2 tablespoons arrowroot
or cornstarch, mixed
with 2 to 3 tablespoons
cold water (optional)
½ cup packed, chopped
fresh basil

Drop the tomatoes into boiling water for 1 minute. Remove and rinse under cold water. Peel off the skins and chop into large chunks. Place in a large saucepan.

Drop the garlic into the boiling water for 1 minute also. It will then peel quite easily. Squeeze the garlic through a press into the pan with the tomatoes. Mash the tomatoes with a potato masher—do not puree.

Add the soy sauce, crushed red pepper, and freshly ground pepper. Bring to a boil, lower the heat, and simmer for 10 minutes. Add the arrowroot or cornstarch mixture, if desired, for thickening. Cook, stirring, until thickened to the consistency you like. Stir in the basil. Remove from the heat and serve at once.

Two-Bean Pasta Sauce

SERVINGS: 10
PREPARATION TIME: 25 MINUTES
COOKING TIME: 45 MINUTES

Serve over your favorite pasta. This also makes an excellent pizza sauce and is wonderful on baked potatoes or mixed with rice. Makes a great Spanish rice if you add peas, corn, and chopped peppers.

8 cups tomato sauce
2 cups tomato paste
2 large onions, chopped
4 large carrots, scrubbed and shredded
One 10-ounce box frozen chopped spinach, thawed and drained
2 teaspoons dried basil

2 teaspoons dried oregano
2 teaspoons garlic powder
6 teaspoons onion powder
One 15-ounce can kidney beans, drained and rinsed
One 15-ounce can black beans, drained and rinsed

Combine all of the ingredients, except the beans, in a saucepan and simmer for 30 minutes. Add the beans and simmer for an additional 15 minutes.

Spicy Pasta Sauce

SERVINGS: 4
PREPARATION TIME: 15 MINUTES
COOKING TIME: 20 TO 25 MINUTES

½ medium onion, chopped
2 cloves garlic, pressed
1 to 2 zucchini, chunked
½ cup water
Three 8-ounce cans tomato sauce

1 teaspoon dried basil
1 teaspoon dried thyme
1 teaspoon dried oregano
2 to 4 drops Tabasco or ½ teaspoon crushed red pepper flakes

Sauté the onion, garlic, and zucchini in the water for about 5 minutes. Add the remaining ingredients and cook, uncovered, over low heat for 15 to 20 minutes.

Marinara Sauce

SERVINGS: 4 TO 6
PREPARATION TIME: 15 MINUTES
COOKING TIME: 1 TO 2 HOURS

Serve over pasta or whole grains, or use in casseroles.

1 onion, chopped
½ pound mushrooms, chopped
2 cloves garlic, finely chopped
One 15-ounce can stewed tomatoes
One 15-ounce can tomato puree
One 15-ounce can tomato sauce

1 teaspoon dried basil
1 teaspoon oregano (optional)
2 tablespoons parsley flakes
2 green bell peppers, coarsely chopped
1 teaspoon Worcestershire sauce

Sauté the onion, mushrooms, and garlic in a small amount of water for 10 minutes. Add the remaining ingredients. Simmer, uncovered, over low heat for 1 to 2 hours, until thick.

Variation: Try substituting fresh herbs for dried in this sauce. They'll really jazz it up. Use 1½ teaspoons *each* of chopped fresh basil and fresh oregano, and ¼ cup of chopped fresh parsley.

Chunky Vegetable Marinara Sauce

SERVINGS: 6 TO 8
PREPARATION TIME: 20 MINUTES
COOKING TIME: 45 MINUTES

1 cup diced green bell
pepper
1 cup diced onion
1 cup shredded carrot
1 cup shredded celery
1 cup sliced mushrooms
3 cloves garlic, minced
1 cup water
One 15- to 16-ounce can
whole tomatoes,
chopped, with
liquid

One 28-ounce can crushed
tomatoes or tomato
puree
¼ cup nonalcoholic red
wine (see Note 2)
1 tablespoon parsley
flakes
1 small bay leaf
¾ teaspoon dried basil
¾ teaspoon dried oregano
½ teaspoon dried thyme
¼ teaspoon dried tarragon

Place the vegetables and garlic in a large pot with the water. Cook, stirring, until slightly tender, about 10 minutes. Add the remaining ingredients and cook, uncovered, for 35 minutes. Remove the bay leaf before serving.

Note: 1. Chop and shred the vegetables in a food processor to save time.

2. Nonalcoholic wine can be purchased at some natural-food stores and some liquor stores.

CHAPTER 10

DESSERTS

The recipes included here are meant to satisfy people raised to believe "dinner isn't over until the dessert is served." (Although there is no reason you must have dessert with your meals.) Many people think of dessert as the richest part of a meal, and the McDougall Program does not violate any present conceptions. Even though these desserts are rich compared to the other recipes in the McDougall Program, they are light-years away from the standard American dessert when it comes to your health.

These desserts emphasize natural sugar, fruits, and fruit juices to provide your sweet tooth buds with plenty of stimulation. Try Apricot Bars, Rice Pudding, Lemon Pudding, Banana Ice Cream, and Apple Crisp for crowd pleasers. Several of the recipes, such as Pumpkin Pie, Lemon Pie, and Persimmon Pie, are made rich by using tofu, which is low in fiber and over 50 percent fat, easily satisfying those of you with a desire for satisfying dinner finales.

Apple Crisp

SERVINGS: 8 TO 10
PREPARATION TIME: 25 MINUTES
COOKING TIME: 30 MINUTES

½ cup old-fashioned rolled oats
½ cup frozen unsweetened apple juice concentrate, thawed
2 pounds Granny Smith apples, sliced

½ teaspoon ground cinnamon
¼ teaspoon ground nutmeg
1 tablespoon whole-wheat pastry flour

Preheat the oven to 425°F.

Coarsely chop the oats in a food processor or a blender. Stir in 1 tablespoon of the apple juice concentrate. Set aside.

Place the apples in a mixing bowl and mix with the remainder of the apple juice concentrate. Add the cinnamon, nutmeg, and flour. Toss to coat.

Place the apples in a nonstick 13 × 9-inch pan. Crumble the oat topping over the apples. Bake for 30 minutes, or until hot, bubbly, and golden brown.

Blueberry Cobbler

SERVINGS: 4 TO 6
PREPARATION TIME: 20 MINUTES
COOKING TIME: 45 MINUTES

⅔ cup whole-wheat pastry
flour
1½ teaspoons baking powder
Pinch salt (optional)

⅔ cup low-fat vanilla soy
milk
3 tablespoons honey
2 cups blueberries

Preheat the oven to 350°F.

Combine the flour, baking powder, and salt. Stir in the soy milk and honey, and mix until smooth. Pour the batter into a nonstick 8-inch square pan. Sprinkle the berries on top. Bake for 45 minutes or until lightly browned.

Date Balls

SERVINGS: 12 TO 15 BALLS OR 12 BARS
PREPARATION TIME: 30 MINUTES
COOKING TIME: 5 MINUTES
CHILLING TIME: 2 HOURS

3 cups chopped dates
1 teaspoon vanilla extract

1 cup water
2 cups puffed rice

Cook the dates, vanilla, and water over low heat, stirring occasionally, until smooth, about 5 minutes. Cool. Add the puffed rice. Form into 1½-inch balls and place on a baking sheet or spread in a nonstick 8-inch square baking pan and refrigerate for 2 hours.

Apple Kuchen

SERVINGS: MAKES ONE 13 x 9-INCH CAKE
PREPARATION TIME: 1 HOUR, PLUS 2 HOURS, 45 MINUTES RISING TIME
COOKING TIME: 30 MINUTES

1 package active dry yeast	¾ cup raisins
6 tablespoons honey	½ cup chopped pecans
1 cup warm water	1½ teaspoons ground
¼ teaspoon salt	cinnamon
1½ cups whole-wheat flour	1½ cups whole-wheat pastry flour

TOPPING

½ cup whole-wheat pastry flour	¼ cup date sugar
	¼ cup chopped pecans
½ teaspoon ground cinnamon	
¼ cup honey	2 apples

Add the yeast, honey, and salt to the warm water and stir until the yeast dissolves. Stir in the 1½ cups whole-wheat flour. Beat until smooth. Cover with a towel and let stand in a warm place for 30 minutes, or until bubbly.

Meanwhile, soak the raisins in warm water to cover for 10 minutes. Drain.

Stir the yeast-flour mixture and add the raisins, pecans, and cinnamon. Mix well. Add the pastry flour a little at a time. Stir until the dough pulls away from the sides of the bowl. Turn out onto a floured board and knead for 5 to 10 minutes, trying not to add more flour unless the dough is too sticky to handle. (It should be soft but not sticky.) Place in a lightly oiled bowl, cover, and let rise in a warm place until doubled, about 1 hour.

Punch down the dough and knead 2 to 3 times. Place in a non-stick 13 × 9-inch pan. Cover and let rise for 15 minutes. While the dough is rising, mix the topping ingredients together. Slice the apples thinly and set aside. Push the dough out to fill the pan evenly.

Layer sliced apples over the dough and sprinkle the topping over the apples.

Preheat the oven to 350°F.

Cover the kuchen and let it rise in a warm place for 30 minutes. Bake for 30 minutes, or until golden brown.

Banana Cake

SERVINGS: MAKES ONE 13 x 9-INCH CAKE
PREPARATION TIME: 30 MINUTES
COOKING TIME: 1 HOUR

2¼ cups whole-wheat pastry flour
2½ teaspoons baking powder
1½ teaspoons baking soda
2¼ teaspoons ground cinnamon
½ teaspoon ground nutmeg
½ teaspoon ground cloves
½ teaspoon ground allspice
¾ cup honey
¾ cup unsweetened applesauce
4 teaspoons Ener-G Egg Replacer, mixed with 8 tablespoons water and beaten until frothy
3 cups mashed banana
¾ cup raisins
¾ cup chopped walnuts (optional—high fat)

Preheat the oven to 350°F.

Mix the dry ingredients together; set aside. Mix the honey and applesauce together. Add the Egg Replacer mixture, banana, raisins, and walnuts. Add the wet mixture to the dry and mix well.

Turn into a nonstick 13 × 9-inch pan and flatten slightly with a spatula. Bake for 1 hour, or until a toothpick inserted in the center comes out clean.

Apple Cake

SERVINGS: ONE 13 x 9-INCH CAKE
PREPARATION TIME: 30 MINUTES
COOKING TIME: 1 HOUR

2½ cups whole-wheat pastry
flour
3 teaspoons ground
cinnamon
2½ teaspoons baking powder
1½ teaspoons baking soda
1 cup unsweetened
applesauce

½ cup honey
4 teaspoons Ener-G Egg
Replacer, well beaten with
8 tablespoons water
2 cups grated peeled apple
2 cups mashed banana
1 cup raisins
1 apple, sliced (optional)

Preheat the oven to 350°F.

In a large bowl, mix the flour, cinnamon, baking powder, and baking soda. In a separate bowl, mix the applesauce, honey, and Egg Replacer mixture. Add the wet mixture to the dry and stir to mix. Add the remaining ingredients, except the sliced apple, and stir until well mixed.

Turn into a nonstick 13 × 9-inch pan and flatten slightly with a spatula. Top with sliced apples and sprinkle with some additional cinnamon, if desired. Bake for 1 hour, or until a toothpick inserted in the center comes out clean.

Pumpkin Cake

SERVINGS: MAKES ONE 13 x 9-INCH CAKE
PREPARATION TIME: 20 MINUTES
COOKING TIME: 1 HOUR

2½ cups whole-wheat
pastry flour
2½ teaspoons baking
powder
1½ teaspoons baking soda
2½ teaspoons ground
cinnamon
½ teaspoon ground
nutmeg
½ teaspoon ground cloves
½ teaspoon ground
allspice

½ teaspoon ground ginger
1 cup unsweetened
applesauce
½ cup honey
4 teaspoons Ener-G Egg
Replacer, well beaten
with 8 tablespoons water
Two 15-ounce cans pumpkin
puree (not pumpkin pie
filling)

Preheat the oven to 350°F.

Mix the dry ingredients together and set aside.

Mix the applesauce and honey together. Add the Egg Replacer mixture and the pumpkin. Add the wet ingredients to the dry and mix well.

Turn into a nonstick 13 × 9-inch pan and flatten slightly with a spatula. Bake for 1 hour, or until a toothpick inserted in the center comes out clean.

Note: For a slightly sweeter cake, increase the honey to ¾ cup and reduce the applesauce to ¾ cup.

Apricot Bars

SERVINGS: 24 BARS
PREPARATION TIME: 15 MINUTES
COOKING TIME: 25 MINUTES

3 cups packed dried
  apricots
Two 16-ounce cans pears, in
  their own juice
1⅓ cups quick oats
1⅓ cups regular rolled oats

1 cup whole-wheat flour
½ cup oat flour (see Note)
1 cup fresh-squeezed
  orange juice
¼ cup honey
1 teaspoon vanilla extract

Place the apricots and the pears and their juice in a saucepan. Cook for 5 minutes over medium heat. Place in a blender or food processor and process until pureed. Set aside.

Preheat the oven to 300°F.

Combine the dry ingredients. Combine the wet ingredients and pour over the dry ingredients. Mix well. Press three-quarters of the mixture into the bottom of a nonstick 13 × 9-inch baking pan. Cover with the apricot mixture. Sprinkle with the remaining topping. Bake for 20 minutes, or until firm. Cool and cut into 24 pieces.

Note: To make oat flour, process rolled oats in a blender or food processor.

Pear Bars

SERVINGS: MAKES 24 BARS
PREPARATION TIME: 40 MINUTES
COOKING TIME: 50 MINUTES

FILLING

One 16-ounce can pears, in their own juice
2 cups chopped dried pears

¾ cup pitted dates
¼ cup minute tapioca
1 teaspoon orange extract

CRUST

1½ cups water
½ cup pitted dates
1½ cups regular rolled oats

½ cup whole-wheat flour
⅛ teaspoon salt
1 teaspoon vanilla extract

TOPPING

1 cup regular rolled oats

Place the canned pears and juice in a blender or food processor and process until pureed. Transfer to a saucepan. Add the dried pears, dates, and tapioca. Simmer, covered, for 20 minutes. Add the orange extract and set aside.

Preheat the oven to 375°F.

Combine the water and dates in a blender and process until finely ground. In a bowl, combine the date-water mixture (reserve ¼ cup for later), oats, flour, salt, and vanilla. Press into the bottom of a nonstick 13 × 9-inch baking dish and bake for 10 minutes.

Meanwhile, toss the remaining rolled oats with the reserved date water.

Spoon the filling over the prebaked crust. Sprinkle, the oat topping over the filling. Bake for 20 minutes, or until firm. Cool and cut into 2-inch squares.

Grape-Nuts Bars

SERVINGS: MAKES 12 BARS
PREPARATION TIME: 5 MINUTES
COOKING TIME: 35 MINUTES

3 cups Grape-Nuts
1 cup low-fat soy milk
1 cup unsweetened
applesauce

1 cup raisins
2 teaspoons vanilla extract

Preheat the oven to 350°F.

Mix all of the ingredients together. Pour into a nonstick 9-inch square baking dish. Bake for 35 minutes, or until firm. Cool and cut into 12 squares.

Oatmeal-Bran Cookies

SERVINGS: MAKES 40 COOKIES
PREPARATION TIME: 30 MINUTES
COOKING TIME: 15 TO 20 MINUTES

1 cup whole-wheat flour
2 cups rolled oats
¼ cup oat bran
¼ cup wheat bran
¼ cup soy flour
1 tablespoon baking powder
1 teaspoon baking soda
2 teaspoons ground
cinnamon
¾ cup honey

½ cup frozen apple juice
concentrate, thawed
½ cup unsweetened
pineapple juice
½ cup raisins
½ cup chopped dates
1 cup chopped walnuts
(optional)
2 teaspoons vanilla extract

Preheat the oven to 350°F.

Mix the dry ingredients together. Mix the wet ingredients together. Add the dry ingredients to the wet ingredients and mix thoroughly. Drop by tablespoonfuls onto a nonstick baking sheet. Bake for 15 to 20 minutes, or until golden brown.

Fancy Fruit Drops

SERVINGS: MAKES 30 COOKIES
PREPARATION TIME: 30 MINUTES
COOKING TIME: 15 MINUTES

2 teaspoons Ener-G Egg
Replacer
½ cup unsweetened
applesauce
1 banana, mashed
½ cup unsweetened peach
juice, apricot juice, or
apple juice
1 cup rolled oats
1 cup quick-cooking oats

1 cup whole-wheat flour
2 teaspoons baking powder
1 teaspoon ground cinnamon
½ cup chopped dates
½ cup chopped dried apricots
or raisins
3 teaspoons vanilla extract
1 teaspoon almond extract
3 tablespoons apple butter

Preheat the oven to 350°F.

Combine the Egg Replacer and applesauce in a bowl. Blend the banana and peach (or other) juice in a blender. Add to the applesauce mixture. Set aside.

Combine the oats, flour, baking powder, and cinnamon in a separate bowl. Stir in the dates and apricots or raisins. Stir the banana mixture into the oat-flour mixture. Add the vanilla and almond extracts. Mix well. Drop by teaspoonfuls onto a nonstick baking sheet. Bake for 15 minutes, or until lightly browned. Remove from the oven. Make a small dent in the top of each cookie and fill with apple butter.

Bread Pudding

SERVINGS: 6 TO 8
PREPARATION TIME: 15 MINUTES
COOKING TIME: 40 TO 50 MINUTES

9 slices whole-grain bread (about 4 cups, cubed)
1 cup vanilla soy milk (see Note)
1 cup warm water
½ cup honey
½ cup unsweetened pineapple or other juice

1½ tablespoons cornstarch or arrowroot
1 teaspoon ground cinnamon
½ cup raisins
¼ cup chopped walnuts

Preheat the oven to 350°F.

Tear the bread into 1-inch pieces and place in a large mixing bowl. Combine the soy milk and warm water; mix into the bread pieces and set aside.

Mix the rest of the ingredients together and add to bread mixture. Pour the mixture into an 11 × 7-inch glass baking dish and bake for 40 to 50 minutes, or until a knife inserted in the center comes out clean.

Note: If using plain soy milk, add ½ teaspoon vanilla extract.

Rice Pudding

SERVINGS: 4

PREPARATION TIME: 10 MINUTES (NEED COOKED RICE)

COOKING TIME: 45 MINUTES

2 cups cooked brown
rice
¾ cup soy milk
¾ cup warm water
½ to 1 cup raisins

2 tablespoons honey
1 teaspoon vanilla extract
2 teaspoons ground
cinnamon

Preheat the oven to 325°F.

Combine all of the ingredients and pour into a 3-quart casserole; cover and bake for 45 minutes, or until set. Serve hot or cold.

Fruit-Rice Pudding

SERVINGS: 4

PREPARATION TIME: 15 MINUTES (NEED COOKED RICE)

COOKING TIME: 30 MINUTES

2 cups cooked brown rice
1 cup crushed pineapple in
its own juice, drained
2 tablespoons raisins
1 banana, peeled and
chopped

¾ cup hot water
¼ cup frozen orange juice
concentrate
1 tablespoon vanilla extract

Preheat the oven to 350°F.

Mix the rice, pineapple, and raisins in a bowl.

Put the remaining ingredients in a blender or food processor and process until smooth. Add to the rice mixture and mix well.

Pour into a 3-quart casserole. Cover and bake for 30 minutes, or until set. Serve hot.

Slow-Cooked English Plum Pudding

SERVINGS: 8

PREPARATION TIME: 1 HOUR

COOKING TIME: 5 TO 6 HOURS IN A SLOW COOKER

The person who sent me this recipe wrote: "This is a wonderful Christmas holiday treat. It is rich with fruit, so we only have it once a year, at holiday time!"

¾ cup whole-wheat pastry flour

½ teaspoon baking soda

½ teaspoon ground cinnamon

¼ teaspoon ground nutmeg

½ teaspoon ground mace

5 tablespoons grated carrot or applesauce

¾ cup fine bread crumbs

1½ cups combination of chopped dates, figs, dried pineapple, dried apricots

½ cup currants

½ cup raisins

½ cup coarsely ground walnuts

Grated zest of 1 lemon

Grated zest of 1 orange

2 tablespoons honey

2 tablespoons molasses

1 teaspoon vanilla extract

⅓ cup brandy (or 1 teaspoon brandy extract)

2 teaspoons Ener-G Egg Replacer, beaten until frothy with 4 tablespoons water

Golden Carrot Sauce (page 340)

Sift the flour, baking soda, cinnamon, nutmeg, and mace into a large bowl. Stir in the grated carrot or applesauce, bread crumbs, chopped mixed fruits, currants, raisins, walnuts, and lemon and orange zests, being sure to coat the dry fruits, currants, and raisins with flour.

In a separate bowl, combine the honey, molasses, vanilla, and brandy. (If using flavoring, add enough liquid—either water or orange juice—to equal ⅓ cup). Beat well. Add the Egg Replacer mixture to this mixture. Combine the liquid mixture with the flour in a larger bowl. (The batter will be more fruit than flour and will be a bit stiff.)

Lightly oil a 2-quart glass bowl that will fit in your slow cooker.

Pour the batter in and cover tightly with a cloth tied with a string. (Leave a loop on each side to aid in lifting the mold from the slow cooker when the pudding is done.) Place 2 cups of hot water in the bottom of a slow cooker. Place the pudding on a rack. Steam for 5 to 6 hours on high.

When done, remove from the cooker, remove the cloth, and cool for 10 minutes in the bowl. Unmold and serve with Golden Carrot Sauce.

Lemon Pudding

SERVINGS: 6 TO 8
PREPARATION TIME: 10 MINUTES
COOKING TIME: 10 MINUTES
CHILLING TIME: 1 TO 2 HOURS

2 cups unsweetened pineapple juice
¾ cup cornstarch
2½ cups apricot nectar
¾ cup honey

½ cup fresh lemon juice
2 tablespoons vanilla extract
1½ tablespoons grated lemon zest

In a bowl, combine ¾ cup of the pineapple juice with the cornstarch. In a saucepan, combine the apricot nectar, the remaining 1¼ cups pineapple juice, and the honey. Bring to a boil. Stir in the cornstarch/pineapple juice mixture and continue stirring until thick and clear. Reduce the heat. Add the lemon juice, vanilla, and lemon zest and stir until blended. Boil for 1 minute. Chill for an hour or two before serving.

Basic Pie Crust

SERVINGS: MAKES ONE 9-INCH CRUST
PREPARATION TIME: 15 MINUTES
COOKING TIME: 10 TO 15 MINUTES, UNFILLED (OR FILL AND BAKE
AS DIRECTED IN RECIPE FOR FILLING)

¾ cup raw cashews or almonds

⅓ cup water

¾ cup whole-wheat pastry flour

Place the nuts and water in a blender or food processor and process until smooth. Transfer to a bowl and add the flour. Mix well until the dough sticks together. Place the dough in a nonstick 9-inch pie plate. Press into the corners and up the sides with your fingers. (Moisten your fingers to keep the dough from sticking to them.)

To use unbaked: Fill and bake according to filling directions.

To use baked: Prick holes in the bottom with a fork. Bake at 350°F for 10 to 15 minutes.

Grape-Nuts Pie Crust

SERVINGS: MAKES ONE 10-INCH CRUST
PREPARATION TIME: 5 MINUTES

This makes a softer crust than the one in the following recipe, and it is also lower in calories.

2 cups Grape-Nuts, crushed (see Note)

⅓ cup water

Mix the ingredients thoroughly. Pat into a lightly oiled 10-inch pie plate.

Note: To crush Grape-Nuts, either place in a blender and process briefly until crushed or place in a plastic bag and gently crush with a rolling pin.

Nectarine-Pineapple Pie

SERVINGS: 8 TO 10
PREPARATION TIME: 40 MINUTES
COOKING TIME: 20 TO 30 MINUTES

CRUST

2 cups Grape-Nuts
⅓ cup frozen apple juice concentrate, thawed

1 teaspoon ground cinnamon
1 teaspoon dried lemon peel

FILLING

One 20-ounce can crushed pineapple in its own juice
2 tablespoons cornstarch
3 tablespoons frozen apple juice concentrate, thawed

1 teaspoon dried lemon peel
3 medium or 2 large nectarines, pitted and cut into ½-inch slices
¼ teaspoon ground cinnamon

Preheat the oven to 425°F.

Crush the Grape-Nuts with a rolling pin or place in a blender and process briefly. Mix all of the crust ingredients in a bowl, then press into a nonstick 9-inch pie plate. Set aside.

Drain the pineapple, reserving the juice. Set the pineapple aside.

Combine the reserved pineapple juice, cornstarch, 2 tablespoons of the apple juice concentrate, and the lemon peel in a saucepan. Stir until well blended. Add the crushed pineapple. Cook over medium-high heat, stirring constantly, until the mixture thickens and bubbles. Continue to cook, stirring, for 1 minute.

Remove from the heat and pour into the crust. Arrange the nectarine slices, skin-side up, over the pineapple mixture.

Combine the remaining 1 tablespoon apple juice concentrate with the cinnamon and spoon over the top of the nectarines. Bake for 20 to 30 minutes, or until the nectarines are cooked but not mushy.

Strawberry-Rhubarb Pie

SERVINGS: 6 TO 8
PREPARATION TIME: 45 MINUTES
COOKING TIME: 30 TO 40 MINUTES

CRUST

2 cups whole-wheat pastry flour

¾ cup finely ground almonds

1 cup unsweetened apple juice, cold

FILLING

2 cups chopped rhubarb

2 cups sliced strawberries

¼ cup fresh-squeezed orange juice

¼ cup Succanat (cane sugar)

3 tablespoons arrowroot

Pour the flour and ground almonds into a food processor. Add the apple juice slowly while processing, until the mixture forms a ball. (It should be sticky.) Refrigerate for ½ hour. Roll out half of the crust to a ⅛-inch thickness and place in a lightly oiled or sprayed 9-inch pie plate. Make strips for the top out of the remaining dough, or roll out a top crust.

Preheat the oven to 350°F.

Mix all of the filling ingredients in a bowl. Pour the mixture into the unbaked pie crust. Cover with either strips or full top crust. Bake for 30 to 40 minutes, until liquid begins to ooze out. Allow to cool before cutting.

Baked Apple-Tofu Pie

SERVINGS: MAKES ONE 10-INCH PIE
PREPARATION TIME: 15 MINUTES
COOKING TIME: 1 HOUR
CHILLING TIME: 1 TO 2 HOURS

1 Grape-Nuts Pie Crust (page 370)
Two 10-ounce packages firm tofu
⅔ cup honey

1 heaping teaspoon ground cinnamon
½ teaspoon ground nutmeg
1 can sliced apples, drained

Preheat the oven to 350°F.

Whip the tofu, honey, and spices in a food processor or blender until smooth as silk. Fold in the apples. Pour into the crust. Bake for 60 minutes, or until firm. Cool. Chill for 1 to 2 hours. Serve cold.

Pumpkin Pie

SERVINGS: MAKES ONE 9-INCH PIE
PREPARATION TIME: 10 MINUTES
COOKING TIME: 45 MINUTES
CHILLING TIME: 1 TO 2 HOURS OR LONGER

2 tablespoons water
One 14-ounce package firm tofu
One 1-pound can pumpkin puree (not pumpkin pie filling)

1½ teaspoons pumpkin pie spice
⅓ cup honey
⅓ cup light molasses
1 Basic Pie Crust (page 370)

Preheat the oven to 350°F.

In a blender or food processor, process the water and tofu until creamy. Stir in the remaining ingredients. Pour into the pie shell. Bake for 45 minutes, or until firm. Chill for 1 to 2 hours or more before serving.

Lemon Pie

SERVINGS: MAKES ONE 10-INCH PIE
PREPARATION TIME: 15 MINUTES
COOKING TIME: 45 TO 60 MINUTES
CHILLING TIME: 1 TO 2 HOURS

6 tablespoons fresh
lemon juice (2 to 3
lemons)
Three 10-ounce packages
firm tofu

1 to 1⅛ cups honey
1 Grape-Nuts Pie Crust
(page 370)

Preheat the oven to 350°F.

Put the lemon halves that have been juiced into a food processor
and chop finely. Add the tofu, honey, and lemon juice. Whip in the
food processor until smooth as silk. Pour into the crust. Bake for
45 to 60 minutes, or until firm. Cool. Chill for 1 to 2 hours in the
refrigerator and serve cold.

Persimmon Pie

SERVINGS: MAKES ONE 10-INCH PIE
PREPARATION TIME: 20 MINUTES
COOKING TIME: 45 TO 60 MINUTES
CHILLING TIME: 1 TO 2 HOURS

2 cups pulped raw
persimmon
⅔ cup honey
Two 10-ounce packages firm
tofu
2 heaping teaspoons
ground cinnamon

¾ teaspoon ground nutmeg
½ teaspoon ground ginger
1 Grape-Nuts Pie Crust
(page 370)
1 tablespoon Grape-Nuts

Preheat the oven to 350°F.

Pull all of the ingredients except the crust and Grape-Nuts in a food processor and whip until smooth as silk. Pour into the crust and sprinkle the Grape-Nuts on top. Bake for 45 to 60 minutes, or until firm. Cool. Chill in the refrigerator for 1 to 2 hours. Serve cold.

Smoothies

SERVINGS: 1 TO 2
PREPARATION TIME: 5 MINUTES

Our children love these for after-school snacks or late-evening snacks.

SMOOTHIE #1

1 banana
½ cup unsweetened apple juice

½ cup frozen strawberries or peaches

SMOOTHIE #2

¾ cup pineapple chunks
½ cup unsweetened apple juice

½ cup frozen strawberries

Place all of the ingredients in a blender and process until smooth.

Fruit Compote

SERVINGS: 4
PREPARATION TIME: 10 MINUTES
COOKING TIME: 4 MINUTES
CHILLING TIME: 2 HOURS OR LONGER

1 cup pitted prunes
¾ cup fresh-squeezed
  orange juice
1 tablespoon honey
Two 11-ounce cans
  unsweetened mandarin
  oranges, drained

Two 16-ounce cans
  unsweetened grapefruit
  sections, drained

Place the prunes, orange juice, and honey in a saucepan. Bring to a boil, reduce the heat, and cook gently for 1 minute. Remove from the heat and cool.

Combine the prune-orange mixture with the mandarin oranges and grapefruit. Stir gently to mix. Cover and refrigerate for at least 2 hours before serving.

Banana "Ice Cream"

SERVINGS: 2
PREPARATION TIME: 5 MINUTES (NEED FROZEN BANANAS)

3 frozen bananas (see
  Note)

⅓ to ½ cup soy milk

Place the bananas and soy milk in a blender or food processor and process until smooth.

Note: To freeze bananas, peel, wrap them in plastic wrap, and freeze for at least 12 hours.

Variations: 1. Add other frozen fruits, such as strawberries, rasp-berries, or blueberries, along with the bananas.

2. Add ½ teaspoon ground cinnamon and ½ teaspoon vanilla extract before blending.

3. For a lower-fat variety, use low-fat soy milk, water, or fruit juice instead of soy milk.

Glazed Bananas

SERVINGS: 6 TO 8
PREPARATION TIME: 10 MINUTES
COOKING TIME: 4 TO 6 MINUTES

⅓ cup frozen orange juice concentrate
6 ripe bananas, peeled and sliced

1 teaspoon vanilla extract
½ teaspoon ground cinnamon

Place the orange juice concentrate in a saucepan and warm over medium heat. Add the sliced bananas and cook for 2 to 3 minutes. Add the vanilla and cinnamon and continue to cook until the moisture is absorbed (another 2 to 3 minutes). Serve warm.

Cinnamon-Apple Chunks

SERVINGS: 4

PREPARATION TIME: 15 MINUTES

COOKING TIME: 6 MINUTES (MICROWAVE) OR 15 MINUTES (STOVE TOP)

Try this on Banana "Ice Cream."

4 apples, cut into bite-size chunks
½ cup raisins

½ cup unsweetened apple or pear juice
Ground cinnamon

Place the apples, raisins, and juice in a microwaveproof casserole. Sprinkle liberally with cinnamon. Cover and microwave on high for 6 minutes, or until tender. If you prepare this on a stove, place all the ingredients except the cinnamon in a saucepan. Cook over medium-low heat for 5 minutes, stirring occasionally. Add the cinnamon, stir, and continue to cook, stirring frequently, until the apples are tender, about 10 minutes.

CONTRIBUTORS

For this cookbook we asked for contributions from many people because we appreciate the wide diversity of people's tastes. A notice appeared in our newsletter asking for favorite recipes, and many people eagerly responded with hundreds of suggestions; indeed, many sent more than one recipe. Other recipes came from people who took our evening health classes and attended the McDougall live-in clinic at St. Helena Hospital in Napa Valley, California. All recipes were carefully evaluated and modified when necessary to fit the principles of the McDougall program.

We believe the response to our request for new ideas for this book was overwhelming because people got a chance to share with others. Although we wanted to use all the recipes we received, we had to choose those that fit best in this cookbook, saving others for our next books. If you have recipe ideas please send them to us:

The McDougalls
P.O. Box 14039
Santa Rosa, CA 95402

If you do contribute, you might find your name in the next McDougall book.

Linda Ayotte
Seasoned Oven Fries

Roberta Wight Beale
Super Soy Sauce

Susan Betancourt
Waffles

Dawn Boyd
DHB's Pasta Fazoola

Bobbie Bramlette
Texas-Style Black-Eyed Pea
Soup

Daria Brown
Basic Cornbread
Marinara Sauce

Louise Burk
Sunny Breakfast Couscous
Cereal

Nancy L. Campbell
Indian Raisin Rice
Tomato-Onion Soup with
Rigatoni

L. Cayard
Whole-Wheat Bagels
Easy Muffins

Teri Crowe
Fruit Carrot-Bran Muffins

Maggie Dunn
Tasty Pasta Sauce

Linda DuPuy
Cilantro Chutney

Karen Engelbauer
Fresh Tomato and Garlic
Sauce

Linda Etherington
Grape-Nuts Bars
Zucchini Bread

Lisa Forrest
Pumpkin Pie
Oat-Turnip Loaf

Riva Gebel
Cuban Black Beans

Marina Gibson
Grandma Gibson's Split Pea
Soup
Curried Red Lentil Soup
Two-Bean and Rice Salad

Sharon Gillespie
Spicy Rice and Beans
Beanburgers
Baked Potato Patties
Cucumber-Dill Crunch
Black Bean Salad
Apple Crisp
Rotini Salad
Date Balls
Blueberry Cobbler

Saundra Guest
Jiffy Vegetarian Posole
Drunken Bean Soup
Tasty Blender Salsa
Spicy Pasta Sauce

Eleanor Guilford
Dutch Vegetable Whip

Martha Gustafson
Split Pea and Lentil Soup
with Vegetables

Lisa Hannus
Tempeh Pâté

Glenda Hazel
Apple Kuchen
Wonderful "Buttermilk"
Pancakes
Basic Corn Muffins

Margaret Hiebert
Oat-Nut Burgers

Maryrose Hopkins
  Holiday Vegebird, Dressing,
    and Gravy
  Whole-Wheat Banana Bread
  Bread Pudding
  Brown Gravy
  Spicy Potato Chunks
  Rice Pudding

Gary and Theresa James
  Slow-Cooked Baby Lima
  Beans

Robert Siegel, the Healthy
Gourmet
  Applesauce-Cornbread Loaf
  Gingered Carrots
  Light Lentil Loaf
  Holiday Loaf
  Carrot Loaf or
    Crispy Burgers
  Vegetable Lasagna
  Peperonata
  Spicy Yam Stew
  Savory Mushroom Gravy
  Strawberry Rubarb Pie

Margi Kangas
  Savory Lentils

Wilma Knox
  Plantation Breakfast
  Indian Lentil Sandwich
    Spread

Xenia Kostrikin
  Macaroni and Cabbage

Bette and Roy Krimont
  Breakfast Polenta with
    Orange-Maple Syrup

Andrea Lemieux
  Layered Vegetable Casserole
  Garbanzo-Broccoli Stew
  Grated Potato Bake
  Stuffed Collard Greens
  Sweet-Potato Puffs

Indian Garbanzo and
  Tomato Stew

Verla Lindstrom
  Sandwich Cheese
  Slow-Cooked English Plum
    Pudding
  Golden Carrot Sauce

Lois MacKenzie
  Tricolor Lasagna
  Mockzarella Cheese

The McDougall Program, St.
Helena Hospital
  Lemon Pudding
  Fruit/Rice Pudding
  Coleslaw
  Broccomole
  Pear Bars
  Herb-Stuffed Squash
  Zucchini Lasagna
  Marinara Sauce
  Garbanzo Shepherd's Pie
  Green Pepper and Tomato
    Teriyaki
  Lentil Chili and Cornbread
    Casserole
  Bean-Corn Enchiladas
  Easy Baked Beans
  Spanish Rice
  Broccoli-Barley Toss
  Kidney-Bean Salad
  Tomato-Rice Salad
  Pesto Pasta Salad
  Chunky Apple Syrup
  Blueberry Sauce
  Peach Sauce
  Strawberry Sauce
  Pineapple-Banana Sauce
  Glazed Bananas
  Tofu Cream Cheese
  Potato Balls
  Country Potato Patties
  Apricot Bars

Marilyn Northcutt
  Nectarine-Pineapple Pie

Nancy Ogle
  Cornmeal Cake
  Quick Bulghur with Pasta

Millie Overholt
  Oatmeal-Bran Cookies

Becky Peckler
  Mediterranean White-Bean
    Soup

Dorothy Pronzini
  Leslie's Soup

The Ramias
  Mama Lucia Marinara Sauce

Mary Reinhart
  Twin Sisters Vegetable Soup

Marilyn Samuel
  Moroccan Chick-peas

Carol Sanderlin
  Spanish-Style Vegetable
    Casserole

Janine Shrader
  Cream of Broccoli Soup

Mrs. A. J. Sorensen
  Apple–Oat Bran Muffins

MaryLyn Spomer, PhD
  Garlic Pasta Sauce
  Vegetable Quiche
  100% Stone-Ground Whole-
    Wheat Bread
  100% Stone-Ground Whole-
    Wheat Dinner Rolls

Sweet Bread
Sweet Rolls
Grape-Nuts Crust
Persimmon Pie
Lemon Pie
Baked Apple-Tofu Pie
Tempeh-Stuffed Peppers
Cajun Black-Eyed Pea Stew
Slow-Cooked Black Beans
  and Prunes
Thousand Island Tofu
  Dressing

Sheila Sterling
  Stuffed Cabbage Rolls

Fred Thornton
  Texas Crude

Ken and Frances Todd
  Stuffed Zucchini

Olivia and Anna Trifiro
  Olivia's Vegetable Pasta

Carol Wayman
  Apple Cake
  Spicy Red Beans
  Spicy Stew
  Green Chili Sauce
  Potato-Corn Chowder
  Hearty Vegetable Soup
  Okra Gumbo
  Banana "Ice Cream"
  Hash-Brown Medley
  Banana Cake

Ann Wheat
  Lentil-Tomato Soup
  Multigrain Hot Cereal

APPENDIX

Mail-Order Houses

This is a partial list of mail-order houses. Contact each for a catalog and ordering information. Ask about their requirements for orders and any extra fees that might be charged. Many offer savings for bulk orders.

Bob's Red Mill Natural Foods
5209 S.E.
   International Way
Milwaukie, OR
   97222
(800) 553–2258;
(503) 654–3215;
FAX (503) 653–1339

Good source of whole grains, flours, beans, pastas, and mixes. Ships minimum order of one full case. UPS within continental U.S. only.

Carr's Specialty Foods
Box 1016
Manchaca, TX 78652
(512) 282–9056

Minimum $25 for credit card order. Ships UPS.

Deer Valley Farm
RD1
Guilford, NY 13780
(607) 764–8556

Minimum order $10. Ships UPS, Parcel Post.

Food Care Inc.
P.O. Box 6383
Champaign, IL
  61821
(217) 687–5115;
FAX (217) 687–4830

**Garden Spot
Distributors**
438 White Oak
  Road
New Holland, PA
  17557
(800) 829–5100;
(717) 354–4936;
FAX (717) 354–4934

Minimum order $25. Ships UPS, USPS.

**Granary Natural
Foods Markets**
1400 Main Street
Suite 207
Sarasota, FL 34236
(800) 274–2749

More than 15,000 items in The National Natural Foods Catalog. Overnight orders.

**Gold Mine Natural
Food Company**
1947 30th Street
San Diego, CA
  92102
(800) 475–FOOD;
(619) 234–9711

No minimum order. Ships UPS, Parcel Post, own trucks. Macrobiotic specialties.

Mountain Art Trading Company
P.O. Box 1037
Fayetteville, AR 72702
(800) 643–8909;
(501) 442–7191

No minimum order. Ships UPS, Parcel Post. Macrobiotic specialities.

Krystal Warf Farms
RD 2, Box 2112
Mansfield, PA 16933
(717) 549–8194

Minimum order 10 pounds. Ships UPS.

Mountain Peoples Warehouse
110 Springhill Drive
Grass Valley, CA 95945
(916) 273–9531
FAX (916) 273–0326

Minimum order $500. Pickup or delivery to Western states only (including Hawaii). Great savings.

Natural Lifestyle Supplies
16 Lookout Drive
Asheville, NC 28804
(800) 752–2775;
(704) 254–9606

No minimum order. Ships UPS, Parcel Post. Macrobiotic specialties.

Nature's Mart
2080 Hillhurst
Los Angeles, CA
(213) 668–0287;
(213) 668–0052

No minimum order. Ships UPS.

Rising Sun Organic   No minimum order. Ships UPS.
Food
P.O. Box 627
Millesburg, PA
  16853
(814) 355–9850;
FAX (814) 355–4871

Simply Delicious   Minimum order $25 for credit cards. Ships
243 A North Hook   UPS.
  Road
Box 214
Pennsville, NJ 08070
(609) 678–4488

Walnut Acres   Organic foods, no minimum order. Ships
Organic Farms   all over U.S. Ships UPS, Parcel Post.
Walnut Acres Road
Penns Creek, PN
  17862
(800) 433–3998;
(717) 837–0601;
FAX (717) 837–1146

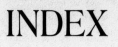

INDEX